Case Studies in Clinical Examination

second edition

Owen Epstein MBBCh FRCP
Consultant Physician & Gastroenterologist
Clinical Tutor & Director of Endoscopy Unit
Royal Free Hospital NHS Trust, London, UK

G David Perkin BA MB FRCP
Consultant Neurologist
Charing Cross Hospital and Hillingdon Hospital, London, UK

David P de Bono MA MD FRCP
British Heart Foundation Professor of Cardiology and Head of the Department of Medicine and Therapeutics, University of Leicester
Clinical Sciences Wing, Glenfield Hospital NHS Trust, Leicester, UK

John Cookson MD FRCP
Consultant Physician & Clinical Sub-Dean (University of Leicester)
Department of Respiratory Medicine
Glenfield Hospital NHS Trust, Leicester, UK

With contributions from:
Neil Solomons MBChB FRCS
Consultant Surgeon in Otolaryngology
Head, Neck and Facial Plastic Surgery
Royal Surrey County Hospital NHS Trust, Guildford, UK

Andrew Robins MB MSc MRCP FRCPCH
Consultant Paediatrician
Whittington Hospital NHS Trust, London, UK

Mosby

London Philadelphia St. Louis Sydney Tokyo

Project Manager: Jane Tozer
Development Editor: Gina Almond
Designer: Paul Phillips
Layout Artist: Paul Phillips
Cover Design: Greg Smith
Illustration: Annette Whalley
Production: Hamish Adamson
Index: Anita Reid
Publisher: Richard Furn

Published in 1997 by Mosby, an imprint of Times Mirror International Publishers Limited

Printed by Lego Print SRL, Trento, Italy

ISBN 0 7234 2579 5

For full details of all Times Mirror International Publishers Limited titles, please write to Times Mirror International Publishers Limited, Lynton House, 7–12 Tavistock Square, London WC1H 9LB, England.

A CIP catalogue record for this book is available from the British Library.

Library of Congress Cataloging-in-Publication Data applied for.

Preface

Despite all the advances in modern investigation techniques, the clinical examination remains the backdrop of clinical practice. It is unlikely that any disorder would escape the scrutiny of a competent history and examination, and the most effective route to investigation is always based on the differential diagnoses developed in the clinic or at the bedside.

The case histories in this book are a companion to the parent textbook, *Clinical Examination, Second edition*, and provide practice in developing diagnostic acumen from the history and examination. Each of the 58 case histories are followed by prompts to encourage the reader to interpret the findings before moving to the next section. The history and examination on each patient is separated from the discussion which allows the reader to compare 'notes' with the expert comments.

Case Studies in Clinical Examination, Second edition is one of four publications in the Clinical Examination compendium. The combination of *Clinical Examination, Second edition*, CD-ROM *Clinical Examination*, *Pocket Guide to Clinical Examination second edition* and this book, *Case Studies in Clinical Examination, Second edition*, offers the complete collection of learning and teaching material for students of clinical medicine.

case 1

HISTORY

Deirdre Symonds, a 70-year-old widow with three children, lived alone and was generally well. She had a substantial circle of friends and was an enthusiastic member of her local Women's Institute. She had been diagnosed as hypertensive approximately 10 years previously having attended her doctor complaining of slight breathlessness and fatigue. Control of her hypertension had always proved difficult and at times her systolic blood pressure had reached 200 mmHg. At presentation she was taking an angiotensin-converting enzyme inhibitor and a diuretic.

A year before, she had noticed an ill-defined blurring of vision on looking to the right. Within a month or so this had become more evident and was now clearly associated with diplopia. Her sight had been assessed at a local eye clinic where it was thought that there was some evidence of a partial weakness of the left medial rectus. The problem was attributed to hypertension and no further action was taken, although a full blood count and her erythrocyte sedimentation rate were checked and found to be normal, as was a modified glucose tolerance test. She began to notice increasing discomfort in and behind the left eye and wondered whether the eye was becoming a little more protuberant. Her vision had remained satisfactory but, if anything, the diplopia was rather more evident and now seemed to be present on forward gaze. In addition, she realised the left upper eyelid was drooping. For approximately 3 months she had noticed an ill-defined numbness in the left forehead but was not confident of any altered sensation in the cheek or chin. Her general practitioner was concerned about the apparent progression of her disability and referred her for a neurological opinion. She had no other neurological complaints and her general health remained satisfactory, although she still had some breathlessness and noticed periodic ankle swelling.

Consider:

- **Where might the lesion be sited on the basis of the history?**

EXAMINATION

On examination she appeared well. Her blood pressure was 190/104 mmHg. She had slight ankle swelling but the jugular venous pressure was not elevated. Heart sounds were normal; there were no carotid bruits and no orbital bruits.

Her visual acuities were 6/6 parts right and left. The left eye was slightly abducted and appeared minimally proptosed. There was a substantial left ptosis. The left pupil was comparable in size with the right but the light reflex (both direct and consensual) was virtually absent. There was no adduction of the left eye and severe restriction of elevation and depression. Some abduction of the left eye was possible but was clearly reduced in degree. When she attempted to look down with the left eye abducted, there was no rotation of the globe. Movements of the right eye were full and the pupil reacted normally. There appeared to be dulling of the cutaneous sensation over the forehead and anterior scalp on the left and possibly over the cheek and upper lip. Sensory examination of the chin was normal. The left corneal response was depressed. The rest of the neurological examination was normal.

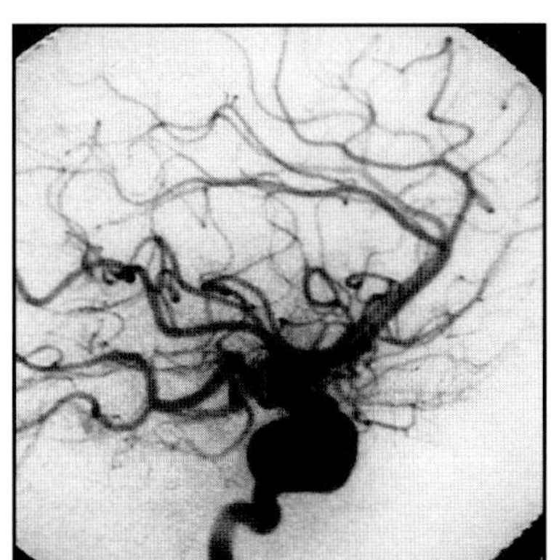

This is the patient's left carotid angiogram.

Consider:

- **What cranial nerves are affected?**
- **Which part of the cavernous sinus is likely to be involved?**
- **Why is the left pupil not dilated?**
- **What is the most likely pathological process?**
- **How would you manage the problem?**

case 2

HISTORY

Edwin Marshall, a 60-year-old man, was brought in by ambulance to hospital complaining of a 30-min episode of severe retrosternal chest pain. He described it as a dull pain that radiated upwards to the jaw and through to the back. He had experienced similar pains on two previous occasions but they were not as severe and had lasted only a few minutes. Previously, the pains had occurred mainly at rest and had no precipitating factors. He had consulted his own doctor concerning the previous pains who had referred him to a local specialist for further assessment. While awaiting for the specialist appointment, his doctor had prescribed a sublingual nitrate spray to be used if the pain should recur. Today's pain had occurred after a large meal. The nitrate spray had eased but not completely relieved, the pain.

The patient denied any symptoms of breathlessness, palpitations or cough. He had recently been experiencing indigestion pains but had not mentioned this to his doctor. He had a history of migraine and depression and had recently been commenced on a tricyclic antidepressant. He had no family history of cardiac disease. He smoked 30 cigarettes and drank a little alcohol each day.

Consider:

- **What are the three major causes of retrosternal chest pain?**
- **What symptoms would help distinguish the causes of chest pain?**

EXAMINATION

A general examination showed the patient to be overweight. He was restless, gripping his chest and complaining of the pain on admission. He was not breathless, pale, cyanosed or sweaty.

His pulse was 70 beats/min, regular and of normal character. His blood pressure was 140/70 mmHg and equal in both arms. The apex beat was not displaced and the heart sounds were normal. No murmur was heard. Breath sounds were regular. Examination of the abdomen was normal, as was a neurological examination.

His electrocardiogram and chest radiograph were normal.

Consider:

- **What physical signs might help differentiate the causes?**
- **What investigation would help make the diagnosis?**

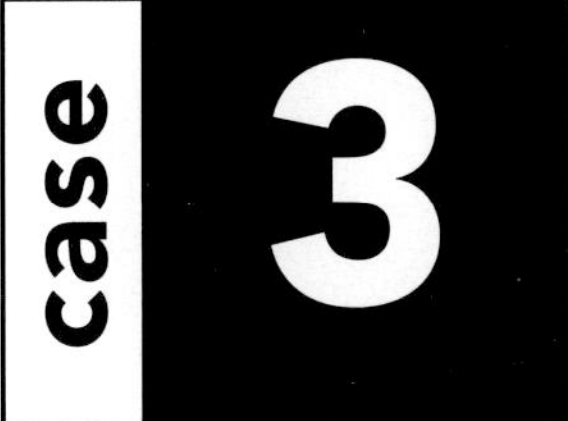

HISTORY

Simone Pritchard, a 48-year-old woman, had always led an active life. She was happily married with two children but was not pursuing a career. Her husband had introduced her to golf 5 years before, since when she had become an enthusiast and had recently been elected the club captain. Her handicap had fallen progressively over the 5 years so that she was now playing off plus 14. She would generally spend approximately 4 h playing a round but had begun to find the last few holes an increasing struggle. Her walking, which she felt had not changed significantly, would begin to deteriorate near the 15th hole. Her legs would start to stiffen and she would find that they felt heavy. Friends would say that her walking appeared laboured and on several occasions she had tripped on divot holes that had not been replaced. If she rested for a while after the round at the 19th hole, her legs seemed to recover. She had recently noticed an occasional stiffness in her legs in bed at night, sometimes causing them to jerk briefly. She denied much in the way of other neurological symptoms but did admit to a change in her bladder function; for some time she had developed increased frequency of micturition, with a sense of urgency and had even been caught short on the golf course. Her general health remained good. She belonged to a private health care scheme and her recent health check had been entirely satisfactory.

Consider:
- **What is the clinical description of this patient's disability?**
- **What is the most likely diagnosis?**

EXAMINATION

On examination she appeared fit and well. The general systems examination was unremarkable. There were no abnormalities in the cranial nerve examination. Upper limb power appeared normal. There was a hint of spasticity in the forearms and the upper limb reflexes appeared uniformly brisk. Upper limb co-ordination and sensation were normal. The abdominal reflexes were absent. There was mild weakness of hip flexion bilaterally but power in the rest of the lower limbs appeared normal. There was definite spasticity in the quadriceps. Both the knee and ankle jerks were brisk, with the ankle jerks tending to spread to the adductors of the thigh. There were approximately six beats of ankle clonus bilaterally. The plantars were extensor. Lower limb co-ordination appeared satisfactory. She was slightly hesitant when identifying small movements of the toes and her vibration sense was absent to the knees. Her gait appeared slightly stiff and she confessed that her walking difficulty was becoming increasingly prominent.

She had already had a full blood count and B_{12} levels measured. Both were normal. She had arranged a computerized tomography scan of the head privately. It was normal.

Consider:
- **Would cerebrospinal fluid examination help in the diagnosis?**
- **What imaging procedure should be performed?**
- **What therapy would control her symptoms?**

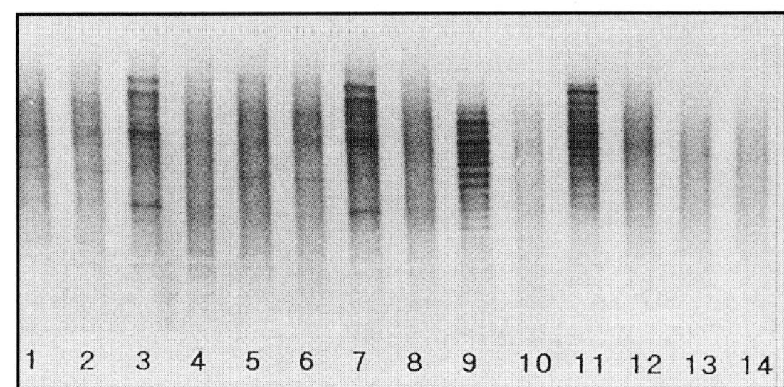

Cerebrospinal fluid electrophoresis was performed as a batch with other samples. The patient's sample is number 9.

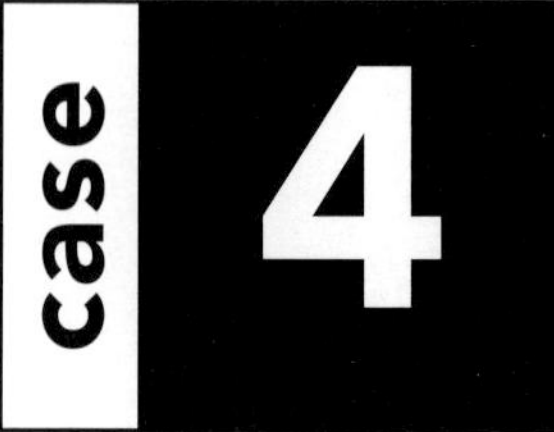

HISTORY

Tiffany Horton, a 27-year-old female research student, had a week's history of chest pain. The initial attack was of severe retrosternal pain that had now eased off but she still complained of a raw feeling in her chest.

The pain was worse if she took a deep breath or coughed. Three months ago she had returned from a holiday spent back-packing in India. She smoked 20 cigarettes a day and was on the contraceptive pill.

Consider:

- **What is the most likely origin of the symptoms?**
- **What is the differential diagnosis?**
- **Is the travel history relevant?**

EXAMINATION

The patient was not short of breath. Her pulse was 90 beats/min and regular, her blood pressure was 100/70 mmHg and her jugular venous pressure was not raised. There were no cardiac murmurs but, on asking her to sit up and lean forward, a scratchy rub was heard on expiration. No abnormalities were detected on examining the lungs. She had some enlarged cervical lymph nodes.

Consider:

- **Do the findings confirm the clinical suspicions?**
- **What are the possible causes of this condition?**
- **What investigations would be helpful?**

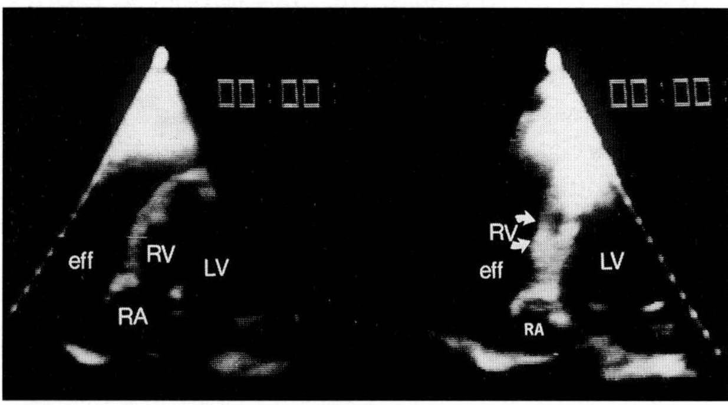

The patient's echocardiogram.

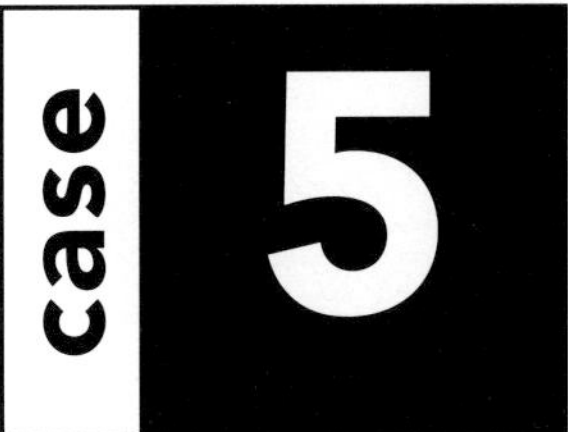

HISTORY

Guy Palmer, a 58-year-old bachelor, had worked in a clerical capacity for the same city firm for over 30 years. He commuted approximately 30 miles every day by public transport, having never learnt to drive. He was abstemious in his habits and, although perfectly amiable at his workplace, had a very limited circle of friends, tending to prefer his own company. His previous health had been good, indeed, few of his colleagues could remember him ever having taken sick leave. Although the firm was fully computerized, he continued to write memoranda and even short letters by hand.

For perhaps six months, it had been noted that his writing had become increasingly difficult to decipher. It was not that his writing was particularly poor, more that the size of the script had become very small at times. He had never had a particularly upright carriage but seemed to be rather more stooped than in the past. His gait had slowed and it was apparent that the morning walk from the station to the office was taking him longer. His voice, never loud, seemed to fade at times almost to a whisper. He was persuaded to have a medical examination, partly because the company was considering offering him early retirement.

He admitted that his physical activities had slowed somewhat but denied any impairment of memory or concentration. He acknowledged that at times he had difficulty getting out of low chairs. He admitted that he occasionally felt dizzy when getting out of bed in the mornings. For some time he had had urgency of micturition and there were times when he had barely escaped being incontinent. He had no other complaints.

Consider:

- **What type of clinical syndrome is suggested by the history?**
- **Are there any features in the history that suggest that this is not idiopathic Parkinson's disease?**

EXAMINATION

On examination his intellect appeared intact. The cranial nerve examination was normal. There was a mild increase in neck tone. There was no limb tremor and power and co-ordination were satisfactory. There was a diffuse, uniform increase in limb tone, predominantly in the upper limbs, which was present even at slow rates of joint displacement. He was bradykinetic, again mainly in the upper limbs and symmetrical in distribution. The reflexes were unremarkable, the plantars flexor. His sensation was intact. His gait showed a reduced arm swing bilaterally. His steps were slightly short and he hesitated a little on turning, although without loss of balance. His general examination appeared satisfactory but his lying blood pressure was noted to be 160/84 mmHg with a standing value (after 1 min) of 140/72 mmHg. He did not complain of dizziness at that time.

Consider:

- **What investigations might assist in establishing the diagnosis?**
- **Will the patient's response to dopa therapy point the diagnosis one way or another?**
- **What advice might be necessary in the light of the blood pressure observations?**

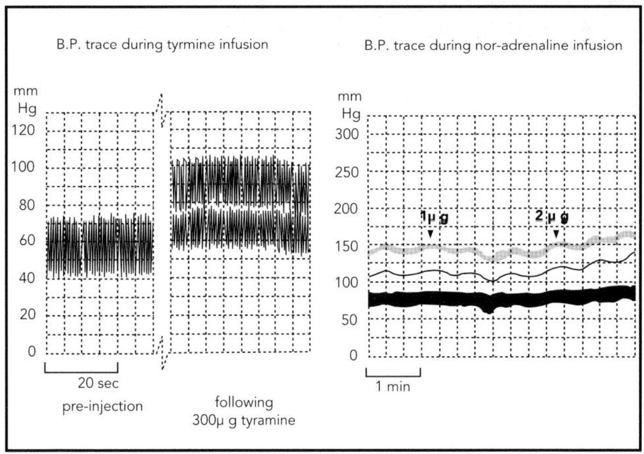

The blood pressure responses to infusion of tyramine (left) and noradrenaline (right).

case 6

HISTORY

Jamie Murdyke, a two-and-a-half-year-old boy, was brought to the Accident and Emergency department by ambulance having had a generalised clonic fit lasting approximately 4–5 min. The ambulance crew had administered 5 mg of rectal diazepam.

His parents were completely distraught but were able to say that he had never had a fit before and that his birth history and previous health were all normal. He had been fully immunised. He had been unwell for the previous 24 h with a mild fever, coryza and cough. His appetite had been poor but he had been drinking good amounts of fluids. His mother had administered paracetamol elixir (120 mg) the day before, the first occasion she noticed a fever.

Consider:

- **What is the most likely diagnosis?**
- **What is the most important differential diagnosis?**
- **What examination findings are of interest?**

EXAMINATION

The boy was asleep on his mother's lap. Both parents were tearful and extremely anxious. The triage nurse's observations included a core temperature of 39.3°C, a pulse rate of 120 beats/min regular, a respiratory rate of 24 breaths/min and an oxygen saturation of 98% in air.

During the examination the following were noted: normal respiratory effort, cool peripheries (capillary refill time 3–4 s), normal breath and heart sounds, a soft abdomen and Kernig's sign. At this point the boy woke up and cried. After a few minutes his mother had comforted him and he was sitting up on her lap and talking and pointing to various features of the emergency room. Examinations of his ears and throat were undertaken, which demonstrated pink tympanic membranes, a red mucous-covered throat without enlarged tonsils and a clear coryza.

Consider:

- **Has the examination confirmed the initial differential diagnosis?**
- **What is the management plan?**
- **What should the parents be told?**

case 7

HISTORY

Rita Lopez, a 45-year-old woman, had recently been in hospital for a hernia operation under general anaesthesia. She was discharged the day after surgery but now, 3 days later, she had been brought back to the hospital as an emergency. Since discharge she had had a slight cold and a severe dry cough. She had, however, been well in herself until earlier that day when she suddenly developed some left-sided chest pain, made worse on deep inspiration. She thought there was a tender area over the site of the pain. She had also coughed up a small amount of yellow sputum with perhaps a streak of blood mixed in. She did not think she was short of breath but had not been exerting herself anyway.

She had been well in the past. There was no personal or family history of thrombosis. She smoked 20 cigarettes a day. She was on no medication apart from hormone replacement therapy for the past 3 months.

Consider:

- **What are the three conditions to consider at this time and why?**
- **What should you particularly look for on examination to decide between these?**

EXAMINATION

She looked well but anxious and had a slight tachypnoea. Her temperature was 37.8°C, her pulse was 100 beats/min with normal character and her blood pressure was 110/60 mmHg. The rest of the cardiovascular system was normal. In the respiratory system, the percussion note was normal and the breath sounds vesicular but there were a few crackles and a pleural friction rub over the site of the pain. No area of discrete tenderness was found. Examination of her legs was normal and the scar was healing satisfactorily.

Consider:

- **How has this examination helped to clarify the initial diagnosis?**

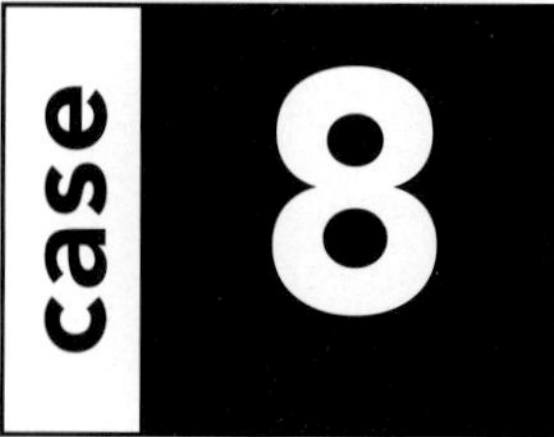

HISTORY

Beth Gubsky, a 23-year-old newly qualified lawyer, visited her doctor complaining of general illhealth and stomach pains. The symptoms had been present for 1–2 months and the patient had initially attributed them to a 'stomach bug'. She described the pains as intermittent and sharp and mainly in the right iliac fossa. The pains were not related to meals or menstruation; they had woken her at night on a couple of occasions.

There was no history of nausea, vomiting or dyspepsia. The patient had noticed her stools to be slightly looser than normal. There was no rectal bleeding. Her menstrual periods were regular. She had lost a little weight recently but commented that she had been put under extra stress with her new job. She had not recently travelled abroad. She had previously suffered from asthma which was well controlled with an inhaler. She was on no other regular medication. There was no relevant family history. She was did not smoke and drank 15 units of alcohol a week.

Consider:
- **What symptoms help decide whether the pain is organic or functional?**
- **Is the position of the pain helpful in developing a differential diagnosis?**

EXAMINATION

The patient looked a healthy, young lady. She was slim. She was not clinically anaemic and there was no lymphadenopathy or jaundice. Chest expansion was normal. Percussion note was resonant and auscultation revealed diffuse expiratory wheeze. A small tender erythematous area was noted on her left lower limb. Abdominal examination was normal to inspection. On palpation there was mild tenderness in the right iliac fossa. There were no masses or organomegaly. Bowel sounds and rectal examination were normal. There were no abnormal findings on cardiovascular or neurological examinations.

Consider:
- **Is there a connection with the painful area on the left lower limb?**

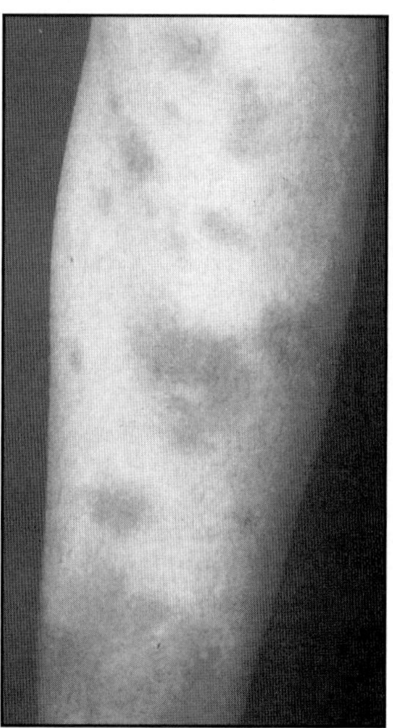

The patient's left lower limb.

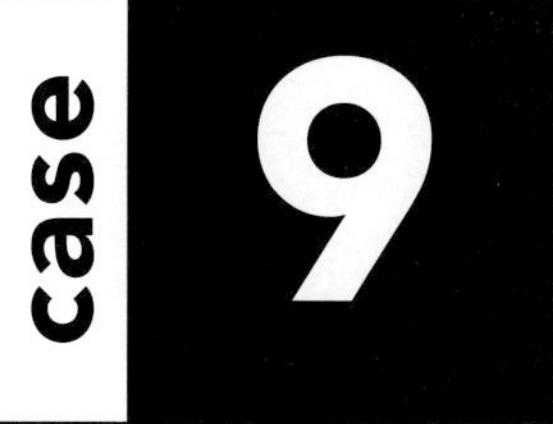

HISTORY

Nicole Yarrish, a 24-year-old single woman, was a trainee opera singer. Her previous health had been good, although she had become thyrotoxic at the age of 20 years. Her symptoms were initially controlled by medication (carbimazole) but eventually she had required treatment with radio-iodine. As a consequence, she now took thyroxine. Her subsequent assessments suggested she was both clinically and biochemically euthyroid. She was aware that there was a family history of thyroid disease. For perhaps a year she had noticed a tendency to fatigue easily, coupled with tiredness. Her general practitioner had found her to be slightly anaemic, of the iron-deficiency type, which he attributed to her heavy periods. He prescribed oral iron but this had no effect. For 3 months she had become worried about her voice. She was now regularly involved in opera performance and was finding that by the end of the opera, her voice was losing its intensity and volume. Luckily, she still sang in the chorus so the problem was not immediately apparent to others. For a month she had noticed a periodic blurring of vision that at times amounted to true diplopia. She could not indicate whether the problem occurred in one particular direction of gaze and insisted that at times it was vertical and at other times horizontal. Occasionally she wondered if her left upper eyelid drooped slightly. Her sense of fatigue had increased and she found her weekend country walk, something she normally enjoyed, increasingly arduous. She had no other neurological complaints. Her general health appeared good. She did not smoke and drank at most 10 units of alcohol a week. Besides thyroxine she was on a mixed oral contraceptive pill.

Consider:

- **What condition could this be on the basis of the history?**

EXAMINATION

On examination she appeared well, although understandably anxious about her condition. The general examination was normal and, in particular, she appeared euthyroid. Her vision was normal. There was a suggestion of a left ptosis that appeared to increase during the course of the examination. She complained of diplopia on right lateral gaze but cover testing did not produce consistent results in terms of involvement of a particular eye muscle. Her jaw and facial muscles moved normally. She had normal palatal elevation and her tongue movements were intact. It was noticeable that by the end of the history her speech had become a little indistinct with a slight dysarthria. In the upper limbs there appeared to be slight weakness of deltoid and triceps bilaterally although the examiner felt her performance was inconsistent. Lower limb power appeared normal as did her gait. Sensation and co-ordination were normal, as were her reflexes.

Consider:

- **What further bedside test could be carried out to add weight to the diagnosis?**
- **What pharmacological test could be of value?**
- **What would be the most important blood test in this situation?**
- **Does the patient need any imaging?**

case 10

HISTORY

Ian Robertson, a 70-year-old man, had a 3-month history of increasing breathlessness. The breathlessness was now brought on by minor exertion such as dressing and he could only walk approximately 50 m before having to stop. His medical history was unremarkable. He said he once took tablets for high blood pressure but gave these up some years ago. He slept badly and found it more comfortable to sleep or rest sitting up. He took indomethacin for arthritis and did not smoke.

Consider:
- **What are the common causes of breathlessness in a man of this age?**
- **Is there anything in the history that points to one of these diagnoses?**
- **Is the medication likely to be relevant?**

EXAMINATION

On examination the patient was breathless from climbing on to the couch. There was peripheral but not central cyanosis. His pulse was 100 beats/min, regular and of small volume. His blood pressure was 150/100 mmHg and his jugular venous pressure was elevated to the level of the ear lobes. Heart sounds were quiet, there were no murmurs and the apex beat was difficult to localise. A few crackles could be heard at both lung bases. There was pitting ankle oedema extending to the level of the knees.

Consider:
- **What is the differential diagnosis?**
- **Do the findings on examination point to a particular diagnosis?**
- **Are there any features that do not at first sight fit with this diagnosis?**

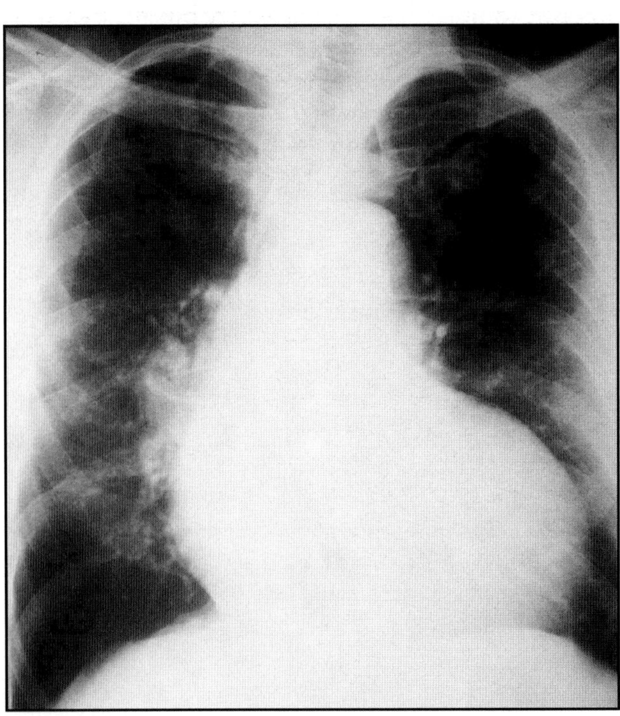

The patient's chest radiograph.

case 11

HISTORY

Brett Campbell, a 25-year-old gay man, had been diagnosed HIV-positive 3 years previously. He had had an attack of *Pneumocystis carnii* pneumonia a year before at a time when his CD4 count had fallen to 10. For 6 months his concentration had started to deteriorate and he had become more forgetful. He had complained of an alteration in his gait. At a neurological examination 3 months before, his doctor had noted a slowing of motor and verbal responses associated with some slowing of saccadic eye movements and broken pursuit movements. The neurologist had made a tentative diagnosis of early stage AIDS-related dementia.

For a month the patient had complained of a dull pain behind the right ear. He had begun to have difficulty in swallowing, with a tendency to choke and splutter when swallowing fluids. He noticed that his speech quality had altered with an element of hoarseness. He felt that his neck was weaker, although he could not specify in what way. Generally, he felt unwell, complaining of tiredness, fatigue and increased irritability.

Consider:

- **Can the previous diagnosis of AIDS-related dementia be sustained?**
- **What clinical syndrome is suggested by the more recent symptoms?**

EXAMINATION

On examination he appeared to have lost weight. His short-term memory was somewhat defective and his mini-mental test produced a score of 25 out of 30. His concentration was erratic and history taking and examination proved difficult. His eye movements were abnormal with broken pursuit movements being particularly evident. His fundi appeared normal. No abnormalities were detected in the fifth, seventh and eighth cranial nerves. When examining the gag reflex, it was noted that he failed to appreciate the pressure of the orange stick on the right but perceived it normally on the left. On phonation, the palate clearly deviated to the left. On inspecting the neck, the right sternomastoid muscle appeared less prominent and the right shoulder slightly depressed. On shoulder shrug, there was delayed elevation of the right shoulder. There was apparent weakness of neck rotation to the right whereas neck rotation to the left was normal. There was some debate about fasciculation on the right border of the tongue but in the end the tongue was thought to be normal. The limb reflexes appeared brisk but the plantar responses were flexor. Limb co-ordination was satisfactory but his gait was slow and rather uncertain.

Formal psychometry was undertaken and supported the diagnosis of an early dementia with some subcortical features. A repeat analysis of his lymphocyte subsets indicated a continuing low CD4 count.

Consider:

- **Does the combination of cranial nerve abnormalities suggest an anatomical site where an underlying pathology may be sited?**
- **What imaging procedure or procedures may be valuable to assess that site?**
- **In the light of the patient's HIV status, what pathological process is suspected?**
- **What is the prognosis for this complication in HIV patients?**

case 12

HISTORY

Sammy Moore, a 6-week-old boy, was sent to a paediatric urgent referral clinic with a history of vomiting after feeds for two and a half weeks, weight loss and irritability on handling.

His parents reported that the pregnancy and delivery were normal and his birth weight was 4.28 kg (>90th centile). He had been jaundiced during the latter half of the first week of life and had been breast fed from birth. He was smiling at 4 weeks and his parents considered his overall development to be normal apart from his poor weight gain which was worrying them.

Consider:
- **What is the most likely diagnosis?**
- **What examination findings are of interest?**

EXAMINATION

On examination his weight was 4.55 kg (<50th centile). He looked thin, dehydrated and hungry. He was not jaundiced or pale. His pulse was 120 beats/min, respiratory rate 30 breaths/min and capillary refill time 3–4 s. The following were normal: heart sounds without a murmur, breath sounds, abdominal examination and tone and cry.

As he appeared hungry and dry, his mother was asked to feed him. After 10 min of breast feeding he stopped feeding. The doctor left the room and returned 5 min later to find the mother in tears and attempting to clean the clinic room floor of a milky nonbile-stained vomit and comfort her screaming infant.

The baby was admitted to the children's ward.

Consider:
- **Has the examination confirmed the initial differential diagnosis?**
- **What needs to be done now?**

The consultant paediatrician comes to review the baby. She has some difficulty in persuading the mother to feed him again. The mother says, 'He will only vomit and get upset again'. The paediatrician says she wants to do a test feed.

Sitting opposite the consultant paediatrician, the mother feeds the baby from her left breast and the paediatrician examines him from his left side, inspecting and palpating from the baby's right upper quadrant. Five minutes into the feed the paediatrician notices visible peristaltic movements in the epigastrium. At 1–2 cm below the right costal margin where the lateral rectus sheaths insert onto the ribcage, deep and medially, a firm swelling can be felt hardening and enlarging.

The paediatrician asks for some blood tests, an intravenous fluid regimen and a surgical referral.

Haemoglobin	**16.3 g/dl**
White blood cell count	**9.8 x 10^9/l**
Platelets	**539 x 10^{12}/l**
Sodium	**140 mmol/l**
Potassium	**2.95 mmol/l**
Urea	**13.6 mmol/l**
Creatinine	**55 µmol/l**
Calcium	**1.14 mmol/l**
Chloride	**80 mmol/l**
Venous blood gases:	
pH	**7.5**
pCO_2	**7.39 kPa**
Bicarbonate	**42.4 mmol/l**
Base excess	**+16.2 mmol/l**

Blood test results

Consider:
- **What do these results show?**
- **How have they become abnormal?**
- **What sort of intravenous fluids should he receive?**

case 13

HISTORY

Monique Spicer, a 63-year-old retired school teacher, visited her doctor complaining of swollen ankles. She had first noticed the swelling 6 months ago, having recently found difficulty in putting on her shoes. She had been feeling tired over the past few years which she had attributed to getting older. Recently the fatigue had limited her in pursuing her hobby of cycling.

She had not noticed any shortness of breath, cough, chest pains or palpitations. She had no pain in her legs. Recently, she had started to itch, especially after a hot bath or getting into a cold bed. She was diagnosed as a diabetic approximately 10 years previously and was currently well controlled on a twice daily insulin regimen. She had taken digoxin for an irregular pulse for many years and used a sublingual nitrate for angina pains occasionally. Her father had died from a myocardial infarct aged 61 years. She drank only at social events and did not smoke.

Consider:
- **What is the differential diagnosis of ankle oedema?**
- **What are two possible causes for her skin itching?**

EXAMINATION

The patient was thin. Her nails were white but she was not clinically anaemic or clubbed. She was mildly jaundiced and had xanthelesmata around her left eye. Her pulse was 65 beats/min, irregularly irregular and of normal character. Her blood pressure was 150/85 mmHg and her jugular venous pressure was not raised. Her apex beat was not displaced. Heart sounds revealed a soft first heart sound and a pansystolic murmur maximally heard at the apex. Respiratory examination showed equal chest expansion, a resonant percussion note and vesicular breath sounds. She had a soft and nontender abdomen. Her spleen was palpable 1 cm below the right costal margin. There was ascites. Bowel sounds were normal and rectal examination revealed only haemorrhoids. She had bilateral pitting pedal oedema. A neurological examination was unremarkable.

Consider:
- **Why does she have white nails?**
- **Why is her spleen enlarged?**
- **How does the history help explain the nature of the underlying disorder?**
- **What blood test confirms the diagnosis?**

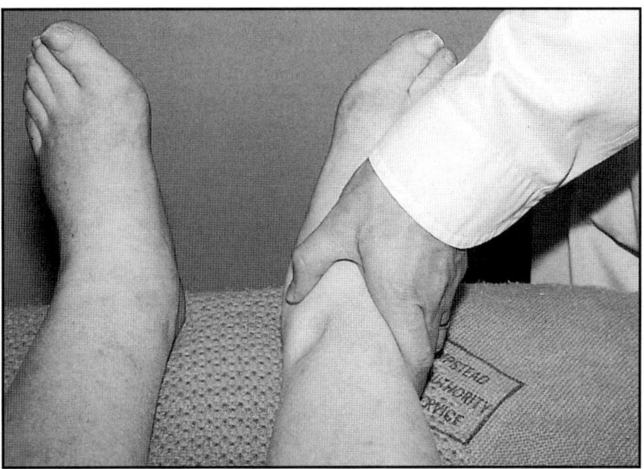

Finger indentation demonstrating oedema.

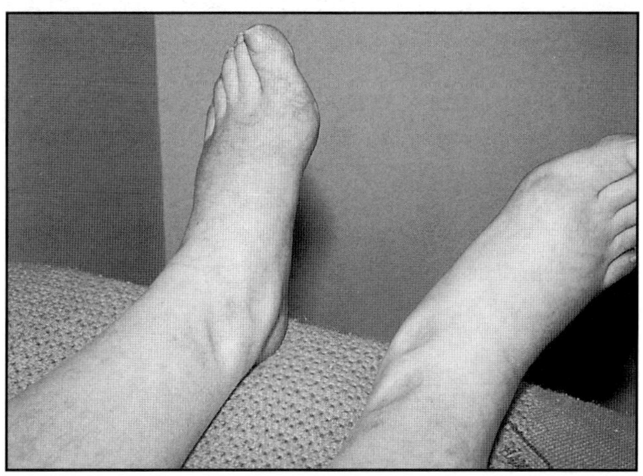

case 14

HISTORY

Richard Chamberlain, a 40-year-old surgeon, presented on 2 January with increasing breathlessness. The previous night he had woken extremely short of breath with a persistent cough and had spent the rest of the night sitting in a chair. He had previously been very fit and had played squash regularly until the beginning of December. He had had a tooth crowned at the end of November. In the week before Christmas he had felt cold and shivery and had a temperature. This had settled with a 3-day course of amoxycillin.

Consider:
- **What are the likely causes of breathlessness in this patient?**
- **What should be thought about the rate of progression of his symptoms?**
- **What may have happened the night before he presented?**

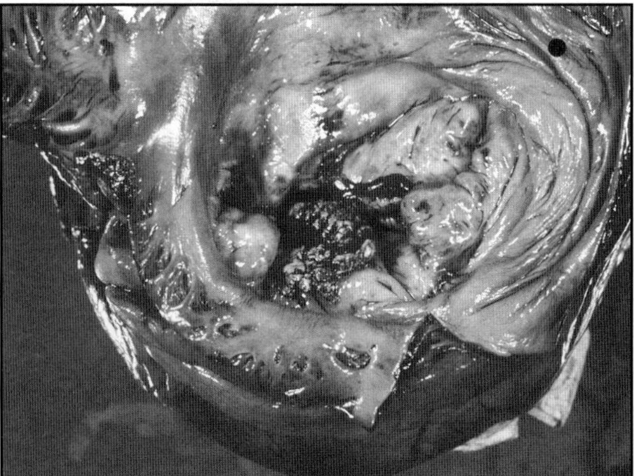

A postmortem photograph (not from this patient).

EXAMINATION

The patient looked generally unwell. His temperature was 38°C, pulse 100 beats/min with a large pulse volume, and blood pressure 120/60 mmHg. The jugular venous pressure was normal. There were bilateral basal crackles over both lungs and a loud early diastolic murmur at the left sternal edge. There were no splinter haemorrhages and there was no enlargement of the spleen. Urine testing, however, showed a trace of blood.

Consider:
- **How has the examination narrowed down the possible causes of breathlessness?**
- **What is the underlying lesion?**
- **What is the cause of the illness?**
- **How should the diagnosis be confirmed?**

case 15

HISTORY

Felix Vazquez, a 70-year-old man, had been mildly hypertensive for several years. His blood pressure control had been satisfactory, using first diuretics, then, more recently, a ß blocker (atenolol). He had sustained a skull fracture at the age of 30 years in a road traffic accident but the fracture was uncomplicated and he had made a complete recovery.

For perhaps a year his wife had noticed a subtle change in his behaviour. He had apparently lost interest in some of his activities. Previously an avid crossword enthusiast, he had neglected to do the crossword on frequent occasions and, on others, had apparently struggled rather more to complete them. He read less often and, although still watching television, appeared to have greater difficulty in grasping current affairs. At times he had been more forgetful in everyday tasks; regularly he would fail to complete all the shopping tasks given to him and frequently when cooking (one of his interests), he would replace items out of position. Rather regularly now he would forget to add salt to his cooking. His driving had become a little more erratic, with a tendency to approach too close to other vehicles and a slowness to react to an emergency. Occasionally he had had difficulty negotiating a route with which he was familiar. In addition to this, he complained of increased tiredness and was tending to nod off each afternoon. His mood had somewhat altered. Previously easy-going, he had become more snappy and irritable. He was less inclined to socialise and when friends visited, he was more withdrawn, becoming increasingly monosyllabic. At times he appeared depressed.

Consider:

- **What is the working diagnosis based on this history?**
- **What underlying pathology is most likely?**

EXAMINATION

On examination his appearance was unremarkable, although he commented on several occasions that he was not really sure why he had needed to come for the consultation. When his wife periodically supplemented the history, he became irritable. His blood pressure was 150/100 mmHg and he was in sinus rhythm. The peripheral pulses were intact, the heart sounds normal and there were no carotid bruits. The routine neurological examination was normal, although at times he appeared rather slow to grasp what was required of him. The reflexes were symmetrical and the plantars flexor. Tests of co-ordination and sensation were normal and his gait was intact.

A brief bedside test of his memory and intellectual function was performed. He was orientated in time, although initially confused the date. He had difficulty in recalling the name of the hospital. He could not remember many details of the recent budget and forgot one of three objects that he had been asked to memorize. When performing serial sevens, he stumbled after the first three answers. He failed with one of the stages of a three-stage command and produced a poor reproduction of a diagram of intersecting figures.

Consider:

- **Has the examination supported the diagnosis?**
- **What blood tests should be performed?**
- **Does the computerized tomography scan help?**

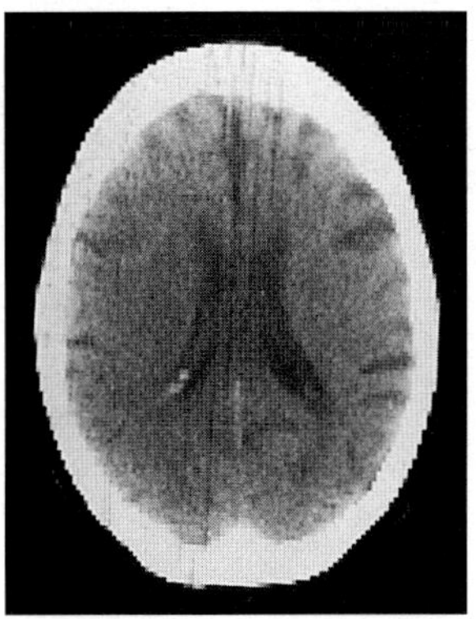

The patient's CT scan.

case 16

HISTORY

Siobhan O'Connell, a 14-week-old girl, was referred to an urgent referral clinic by her general practitioner because she had been screaming constantly for the past 2 nights.

Her mother was worried. The baby was the youngest of four children; her mother had also adopted two other children as infants. The doctor described her as 'an experienced and sensible' mother. The doctor could find no adverse features on examination.

The baby was born after a completely normal pregnancy and delivery. She was breast and bottle fed on demand and described as 'colicky' during the first 2 months. She had normal development and growth (along 10th centile for weight, length and head circumference since birth). She was fully immunised so far. The mother had not been aware of any fever, vomiting, diarrhoea, coryza or rash.

The mother said that when the baby screamed, she was inconsolable for 5–20 min, then she became exhausted and fell asleep, only to start up again if disturbed. There might be 10–12 episodes a night. The mother was adamant that the cry was different from that caused by the 'colic'.

Consider:
- **What is the most likely diagnosis?**
- **What is the differential diagnosis?**
- **What examination findings are of interest?**

EXAMINATION

The baby's length, weight and head circumference were as noted on the 10th centile. She seemed well and even smiled. She had no fever or rash. She had a normal fontanelle, pulse, perfusion and respiration. The chest was clear with normal heart sounds and no murmur and the abdomen soft with no palpable masses. Neurology was normal; she handled well and was active and alert.

On examination the mother looked pale, drawn and tired.

Consider:
- **Has the examination confirmed the initial differential diagnosis?**
- **What is the management plan?**

As a result of the mother being so adamant there was a problem, despite an inconclusive examination, the baby was admitted to the children's ward for observation and a few basic tests.

The nurses noted that she did tend to scream occasionally for no clear reason. All ward observations were normal. The senior nurses said she sounded 'colicky'. A bag urine sample was sent for culture and the baby was discharged with an arrangement to see her in the clinic the next week. The mother was still worried, although she was happy to go home having had at least one night of sleep.

The urine grew more than 100 000 *Escherichia coli* and pus cells were seen on microscopy. The baby was recalled and a repeat clean catch urine was also positive for infection. She was given a course of antibiotics.

Follow-up urine cultures were sterile and she was continued on prophylactic trimethoprim and arrangements were made for radiological imaging of her renal tract.

case 17

HISTORY

Janet Silverstein, a 35-year-old woman, had a bilateral watery nasal discharge (rhinorrhoea). The discharge was present all year round, although it was worse in the spring. She had a poor sense of smell and had had no response to inhaled nasal steroids.

Six years before presentation she had some form of nasal surgery but she could not remember what that was.

She had no history of asthma or aspirin sensitivity.

Consider:
- **Does she have any known allergies?**
- **What examinations should be carried out?**
- **What is the likely diagnosis?**

EXAMINATION

A watery discharge was present at the anterior nares. On inspecting both nasal cavities, nasal polyps were found. Examination of the oral cavity and pharynx revealed no abnormality but polyps were seen in the choanae on examination of the postnasal space.

Consider:
- **Has the examination helped clarify the initial differential diagnosis?**
- **Are there any predisposing factors from the history?**
- **Are there any complications?**

case 18

HISTORY

Maria Muller, a 51-year-old secretary, complained of difficulty swallowing. The symptom had been first noticed 9 months previously but had only become troublesome for the past couple of months. She noticed that solids were more problematic than liquids. A drink of water was sometimes required to help in the swallowing of meat and dry foods such as bread. She pointed to the lower end of the sternum to show where she felt the food sticking. The problem was intermittent but becoming more frequent. She had no pain on swallowing and had lost no weight. She had no cough.

Her appetite was good and there was no history of nausea, vomiting or abdominal pain. She had a 1-year history of indigestion treated by medicines purchased from her local chemist. Last winter she had noticed her hands going cold and blue when outside. Recently, her typing had slowed down because of stiff fingers. She had a history of an appendicectomy when aged 25 years and a cholecystectomy aged 48 years. She was on no regular prescribed medication. There was no family history of swallowing problems but her father had a history of a stomach ulcer. She did not drink alcohol and had given up smoking 3 years ago.

Consider:
- **What is the differential diagnosis of dysphagia?**
- **Is there a link between her presenting symptoms and the cold sensitivity and stiffness of the fingers?**

EXAMINATION

The patient was slender but not cachectic. There was no clinical evidence of anaemia, jaundice, clubbing or lymphadenopathy. Her nails were normal and her hands were warm and of normal colour. She had skin tethering over the dorsum of her hands. Her radial pulse was of normal character and 70 beats/min. There were a few telangiectasiae. Her blood pressure was 110/65 mmHg. Heart sounds were normal. Respiratory examination showed normal expansion, a resonant percussion note and vesicular breath sounds. Abdominal examination was normal other than two operative scars. Cranial nerve examination was entirely normal, as was her peripheral nervous system.

Consider:
- **What syndrome does she have?**
- **How does it affect swallowing?**
- **What radiograph might be helpful?**
- **What other diagnostic tests would be useful?**

case 19

HISTORY

Bill Carter, a 45-year-old man, had been admitted to hospital by his general practitioner one cold night in January in the middle of an influenza epidemic. He had noticed nothing amiss until 5 days previously when he, like other members of his family, 'went down' with 'flu. He had fever, cough and muscular aching. After approximately 2 days he began to recover but then approximately 24 h before admission he became worse again with recurrence of fever, more cough, yellow sputum tinged with blood and then some right-sided chest pain, worse on deep breathing and coughing. He had also been short of breath.

He denied any previous illness but his wife, who was sitting beside him, confirmed that he had had a cough for as long as she had known him but that he had refused to see a doctor about this. On direct questioning, the patient admitted that this was the case but because he had always had this he regarded it as normal; in any event he smoked 10 cigarettes a day. He remembered that he had to attend hospital as a child for some 'breathing exercises' but could recall nothing further of this. He had had no previous breathlessness or wheeze.

Consider:

- **What is the most likely cause of his most recent symptoms and why?**
- **What is the likely underlying problem?**
- **What examination should be carried out?**

EXAMINATION

The patient appeared flushed and unwell. There were Herpes simplex lesions around his mouth. His temperature was 38.5°C, pulse 105 beats/min and blood pressure 110/75 mmHg. Apart from the tachycardia, the cardiovascular system was normal. In the respiratory system examination, the main findings were in the right chest where the expansion on that side was reduced, the percussion note dull and there was bronchial breathing and whispering pectoriloquy. There was also a pleural friction rub over the site of the pain. At the left base there was a localised area of coarse crackles that did not shift on coughing.

Consider:

- **How has the examination helped to clarify the initial diagnosis?**
- **What is the significance of the findings at the left base?**
- **What are the likely organisms causing this patient's symptoms?**

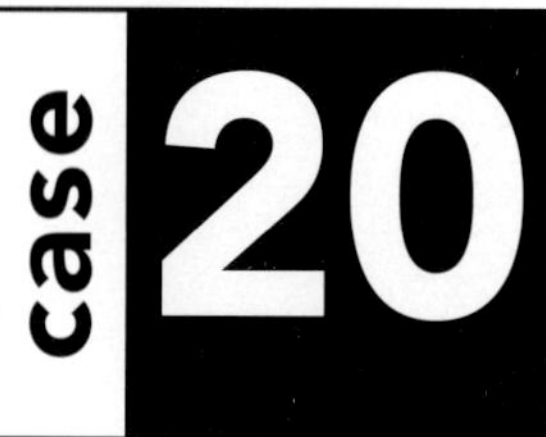

HISTORY

Gurdeep Gill, a 77-year-old Asian gentleman sought medical attention. He complained of a recent history of fevers. The fevers began a week ago and had become associated with feelings of malaise and bone and joint aches. He had recently been to the local hospital outpatient department for his regular blood pressure 'check up'. At that time, he had complained of a cough productive of green sputum and some breathlessness. The attending doctor had noted some crepitations at the base of his left lung, a normal blood pressure and a murmur suggestive of mitral regurgitation. The doctor at that time had prescribed a penicillin for a presumed chest infection.

After this visit, the patient had begun to feel unwell. There had been a recent influenza outbreak. He had a past history of hypertension and pulmonary tuberculosis treated at the age of 50 years. He smoked five cigarettes a day and drank no alcohol.

Consider:
- **What is the differential diagnosis of his fever?**
- **What is the significance of the other presenting symptoms?**

EXAMINATION

Initial examination found the patient to be a thin, elderly and ill-looking man. He had a fever, temperature 38°C. There was no evidence of jaundice, anaemia, cyanosis, clubbing or lymphadenopathy. There was no rash. His pulse was 90 beats/min, regular and of normal character. His blood pressure was 150/90 mmHg. His apex beat was not displaced. Heart sounds revealed a soft ejection systolic murmur at the left sternal edge which did not radiate. His jugular venous pressure was raised by 2 cm. Chest expansion was normal, percussion note was resonant and auscultation revealed diffuse expiratory wheeze and bilateral fine basal crepitations. Abdominal and neurological examinations were normal.

Consider:
- **Which clue in the history and examination provides a high index of suspicion?**
- **What is the likely causative organism?**
- **What other physical signs would you look for?**
- **How would you confirm the diagnosis?**

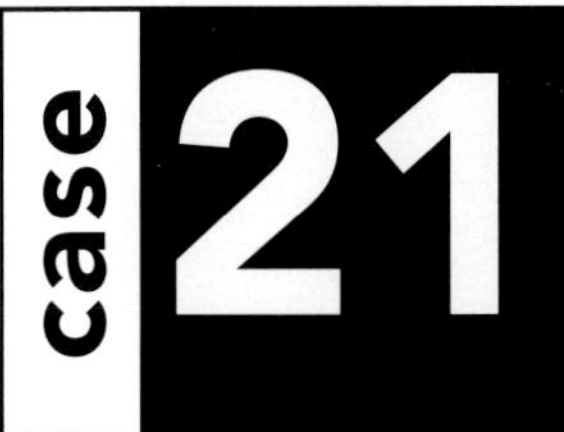

HISTORY

Edward Forshaw-Smyth, a 19-year-old man, was fit and healthy. He had had no significant previous illness. He was an avid sportsman and regularly played cricket and rugby. Although normally a centre, he had been persuaded to move to loose forward on the previous day. The match had been fairly uneventful but, towards the end, the scrum had collapsed causing his neck to be twisted painfully. He was able to finish the game but continued to complain of neck pain during the evening and had to take aspirin in order to sleep.

The pain was still present the next day. Around midday, he suddenly developed intense vertigo and vomited profusely. He decided to go back to bed and slept for a short period. On waking, the vertigo was still present, although less severe and he began to have incessant hiccoughs. He tried various manoeuvres to eliminate the hiccoughs and was disconcerted to find that if he tried to swallow fluids, he began to choke. He decided to telephone his parents, whom he was expecting to see that afternoon. By now he was experiencing an intense pain behind the left ear, different from the neck pain of the previous day. He found he was unsteady as he walked to the telephone and realised he was slurring his words when he spoke to his mother. His mother became alarmed and called an ambulance. There was not a great deal of additional history to give to the casualty officer, although the patient now felt that sensation was defective on the left side of his face.

Consider:
- **Which part of the nervous system has been affected?**
- **What underlying process may have caused this damage?**

EXAMINATION

On examination the patient was alert. His blood pressure was 118/64 mmHg and he was in sinus rhythm. Heart sounds were normal and the peripheral pulses intact. He appeared to be tender over the left side of the neck and was reluctant to rotate his neck to either side.

The left pupil was slightly smaller than the right and there was a hint of a left ptosis. He had nystagmus on right lateral gaze with the fast phase to the right. He had some blunting of pin prick over the left face in all three divisions. He was dysarthric and was still hiccoughing. His palate deviated to the right. His left arm and leg were ataxic but power appeared intact. The limb tone was normal and his reflexes were symmetrical. The right plantar was flexor, the left extensor. When he tried to stand, he immediately fell to the left. Limb sensation to light touch and vibration were normal but he had altered pin prick and temperature sensation on the right leg. This ascended on to the trunk to a variable level on the chest wall.

Consider:
- **Has the examination pin-pointed the site of the lesion more accurately?**
- **What is the usual pathological basis for this syndrome?**
- **What investigations would be appropriate?**

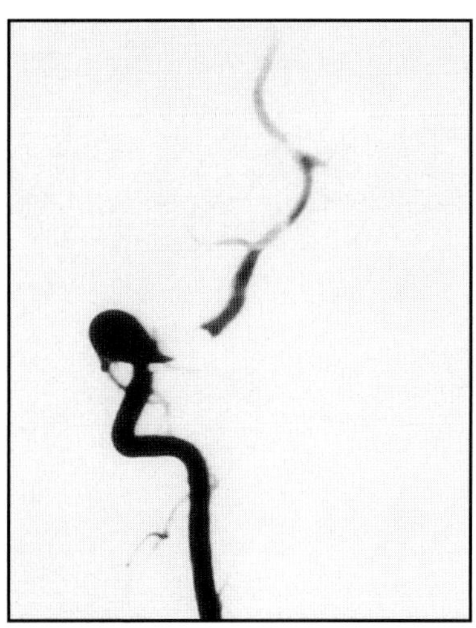

This is the patient's left vertebral angiogram.

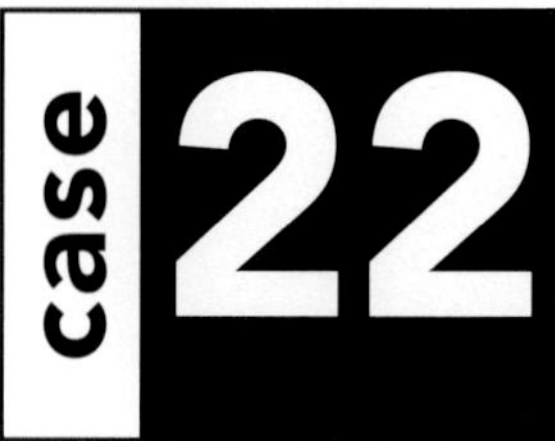

HISTORY

Precious Williams, a three-and-a-half-year-old girl was admitted at 3.30 a.m. to the Accident and Emergency department with a generalised seizure. She had been sleeping in her parents bed when her father woke up to find her hot and having a series of three generalised clonic convulsions lasting approximately 5 min with only 2–3 min in between. He called an ambulance and tried to cool her down. When the paramedics arrived she had further seizures and was given 5 mg of rectal diazepam.

Her mother said she had been pyrexial during the previous 2 days and had been vomiting and refusing feeds the evening before admission. There was no medical history of note and she had been fully immunised.

Consider:
- **What is the most likely diagnosis?**
- **What is the most important differential diagnosis?**
- **What examination findings are of interest?**

EXAMINATION

The baby was drowsy, vocalising inappropriately and pyrexial (39.1°C) without a rash. Her pulse was 110 beats/min regular and blood pressure was 110/60 mmHg. She had a capillary refill time of 2 s. The chest was clear with no respiratory distress, the abdomen soft, Kernig's sign positive and the pupils equal and reacting. The throat was red, the coryza clear and the ear drums pink.

Consider:
- **Has the examination confirmed the initial differential diagnosis?**
- **What tests should be performed?**
- **What is the management plan?**

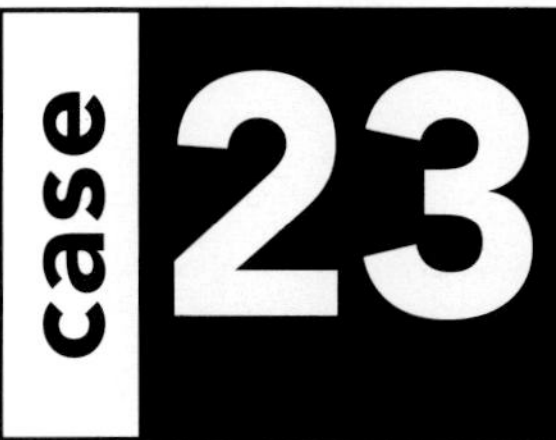

HISTORY

David Homanin, a 65-year-old man, had a swelling in the right jugulodigastric area of the neck. The swelling was not painful but had gradually increased in size over the past 4 weeks.

He had a history of smoking 20 cigarettes a day and he also drank over 20 units of alcohol a week. He had pain on swallowing and had lost 7 kg in weight over the past 4 weeks.

Consider:
- **What is the likely origin of the symptoms and why?**
- **What is the most likely diagnosis and why?**
- **What examinations should be carried out?**

EXAMINATION

The mouth and throat revealed a poor state of oral and dental hygiene. There was significant gum disease and the teeth were carious. The tongue was furred. Indirect mirror examination of the hypopharynx and larynx revealed an ulcer in the right piriform fossa. There was no evidence of any other specific disease focus in the upper aerodigestive tract.

Palpation of the neck confirmed the presence of a 4 cm firm, immobile lymph node in the right jugulodigastric region.

Consider:
- **Are there any predisposing factors in the history?**
- **Has the examination given the diagnosis?**
- **Are any further investigations necessary?**

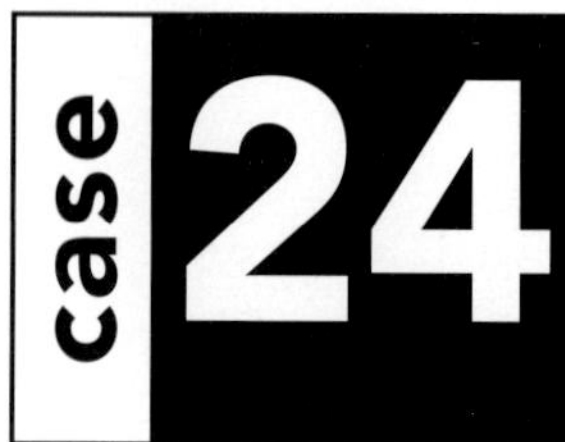

HISTORY

Chuck Stover, a 43-year-old unemployed manual labourer, walked into the emergency department of his local hospital complaining that his eyes had turned yellow. He was a rather vague historian as was his accompanying friend. People had commented that his eyes were yellow 1–2 weeks previously. He had more recently experienced some symptoms of generally feeling unwell, nausea and some diarrhoea. He had been opening his bowels 2–3 times a day; his stools had been loose with a normal colour. He had not noticed any rectal bleeding. Three weeks previously he had attended the same emergency department where erythromycin had been prescribed for a upper respiratory tract infection. Studying his hospital records revealed he had no history other than a road traffic accident requiring some orthopaedic surgery some 10 years ago. At that time he had received a blood transfusion. He denied any previous intravenous drug use and had not recently travelled abroad. He had no family or contact history of jaundice. He smoked between 20 and 30 cigarettes a day and had been drinking alcohol more heavily recently after the breakdown of his marriage.

Consider:
- **What might be causing the jaundice?**
- **Why might he be confused?**

EXAMINATION

The patient was agitated, unkempt and uncooperative during the examination. He was slightly confused and had a fine tremor at rest. He was tattooed and icteric. Temperature was 37.5°C. There were no peripheral stigmata of chronic liver disease. Abdominal examination revealed hepatomegaly to 4 cm below the costal margin. There was no spleen or other organ palpable. There were no clinical signs of ascites. Auscultation revealed a quiet hepatic bruit. Rectal examination was normal. He was not oedematous. Examination of his chest only revealed some transmitted upper airways sounds. There were no abnormal findings in his cardiovascular system. There were no focal neurological signs to explain his confusion.

Consider:
- **How does the examination help to refine the differential diagnosis?**
- **Why is there a tremor?**
- **What condition does the neurological examination exclude?**
- **What are the causes of an hepatic bruit?**

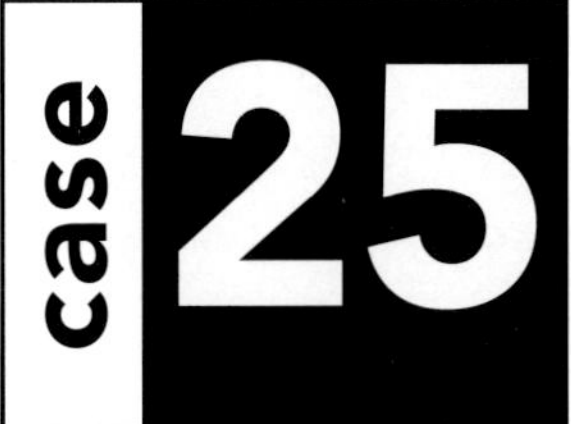

HISTORY

Linda-May Fisher, a 68-year-old woman, was in reasonably good health, although she had been troubled by osteoarthritis of the right knee for some time. This caused her pain and interfered to some extent with her walking. She had had episodic neck pain for some years but a year previously, while attending her yoga class, she had developed a more acute and intense pain in the neck which had radiated to the posterior aspect of the right upper arm. She had seen her general practitioner who advised analgesics and a soft collar. She decided to visit an osteopath. The osteopath seemed to help the problem, although she did notice, after her third visit, some paraesthesiae in the right index finger. Eventually the pain resolved, although the paraesthesiae persisted to some degree.

Over the next year the pain recurred periodically, although never to the same degree and usually responded to analgesics. She also noticed, at times, a sense of twitching in the right arm which seemed to be confined to the back of the upper arm. She was more concerned, however, about her walking. It was not just that she still had a painful right knee but that both her legs felt slightly stiff and heavy. Friends commented that she seemed to drag them and would good-naturedly tell her to hurry up.

She had periodic headaches and had slight impairment of her central vision diagnosed as a form of familial macular degeneration. She lived with her husband and had close contact with her three children. She was trying to give up smoking and had reduced her consumption to five cigarettes a day. She did not drink alcohol and was on no medication except for occasional analgesics.

Consider:

- **What is the likely basis for the long-standing symptoms in the right arm?**
- **What is the basis for the more recent lower limb syndrome?**

EXAMINATION

Her general systems examination was normal, although osteoarthritic changes were evident in the right knee with slight loss of muscle bulk in right quadriceps. Her visual acuities were 6/12 bilaterally with correction and there was evidence of macular degeneration. The rest of the cranial nerve examination was normal. Her neck movements were slightly restricted and a little uncomfortable. In the upper limbs there was mild weakness of right triceps and possible weakness of the small hand muscles on the right. Fasciculation was noted in right triceps. The biceps and supinator reflexes were absent on the right but associated with brisk finger flexion. The triceps jerks were unremarkable but the finger jerks were prominent bilaterally. Tone was normal. There was some cutaneous loss of sensation in the right index finger. The legs appeared slightly spastic with brisk reflexes. The right planter was equivocal. There was a suggestion of hip flexion weakness bilaterally. Proprioception was defective in the toes. Limb co-ordination was intact. Her gait appeared slightly spastic.

Consider:

- **What segmental level is suggested by the upper limb motor findings?**
- **What segmental level is suggested by the upper limb sensory findings?**
- **What is the interpretation of the upper limb reflex changes?**
- **How should this patient be investigated?**

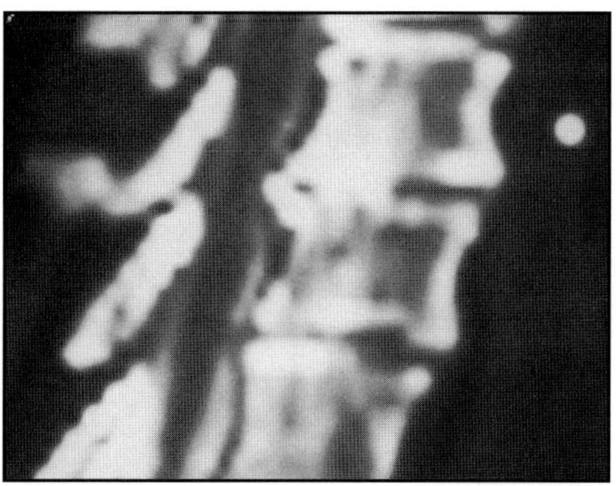

This is the patient's cervical CT myelogram.

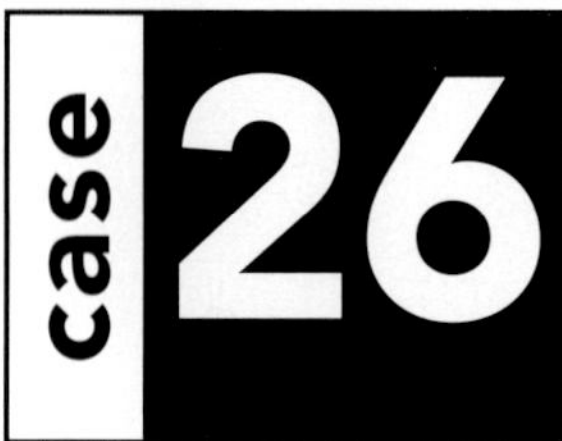

HISTORY

Clark Parker, a 67-year-old retired journalist, complained of itching. The itch had been getting progressively worse over the past 6 months and affected his whole body. He had noticed no rashes. He had been otherwise feeling relatively well. He noticed that the itch was worse after a hot bath and he had taken to bathing in cooler water. On direct questioning he did admit to some tiredness and the occasional dizzy spell. He had not been in contact with anyone with any skin complaint to the best of his knowledge.

The patient had a history of atopy and he had suffered from mild asthma and eczema in his earlier years. He had hypertension that was well controlled by a ß-blocker. There was no recent change in medication. He had a history of hyperthyroidism treated with radioactive iodine some 10 years ago. He had been on the same dose of digoxin for the past 2 years. He smoked 10 cigarettes a day and drank alcohol rarely.

Consider:

- **What are the systemic disorders which cause skin itching?**

EXAMINATION

The patient was overweight. He was plethoric. There was no evidence of cyanosis, clubbing, anaemia or lymphadenopathy. He was comfortable at rest. There was no tremor. His pulse was 72 beats/min and normal. There were no murmurs to be heard and his blood pressure was normal. Respiratory examination was unremarkable. There was a 1–2 cm hepatosplenomegaly. Neurological examination was also normal. On fundoscopy, the retinal veins appeared dilated and 'sausage' shaped.

Consider:

- **What physical signs suggest the cause of his itching?**
- **Which negative physical signs make a clinical diagnosis?**
- **What complications occur?**
- **How is the diagnosis confirmed?**

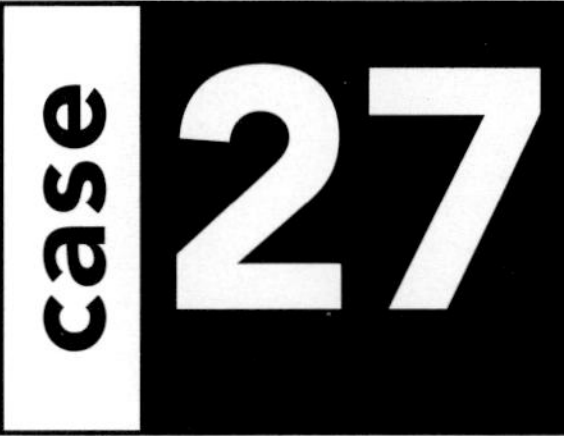

HISTORY

Bobby Elliot, an 8-year old-boy, had a swelling in the midline of the neck. The swelling had been noticed for 4 months. It was not tender.

He was generally fit and well. He had no problem swallowing. He had not noticed any other lumps and bumps around the head and neck.

Consider:
- **What diagnosis is most likely and why?**
- **What examination and investigations should be carried out?**

EXAMINATION

The boy appeared well with no evidence of weight loss or anaemia. Examination of the mouth and throat revealed no abnormality. Palpation of the neck revealed a 2 cm mobile mass just to the left of the midline between the hyoid bone and the thyroid cartilage. The mass was nontender and mobile. There were no other masses palpable in the neck. Both axillae and groins were clear of lymphadenopathy. On protrusion of the tongue, the mass was seen to move superiorly in the neck.

Consider:
- **Does the examination give the diagnosis?**
- **Are any investigations necessary?**

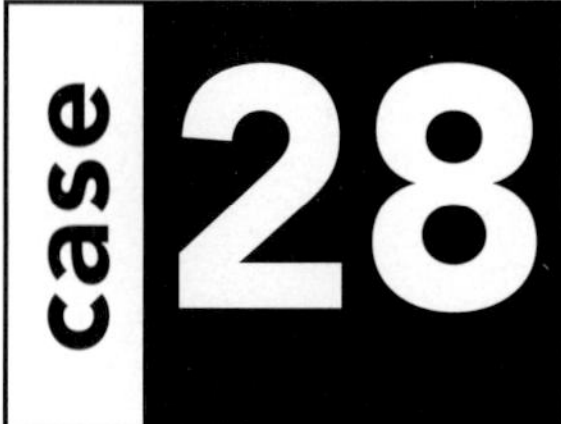

HISTORY

Rita Saunders, a 58-year-old widow, presented with palpitations and ankle swelling after a trip to Florida. The palpitations had started suddenly and continued ever since. Initially she had felt very breathless but, after Emergency Room treatment in the USA, she felt improved. She had lost 2 kg in weight since her husband's death 6 months ago. She admitted to drinking four or five vodkas a night at weekends. Her current medication consisted of low dose aspirin and digoxin which had been given to her in the USA.

Consider:

- **What are the common causes of palpitation?**
- **How does the history help to distinguish between them?**
- **Does the history give any clues about predisposing factors?**

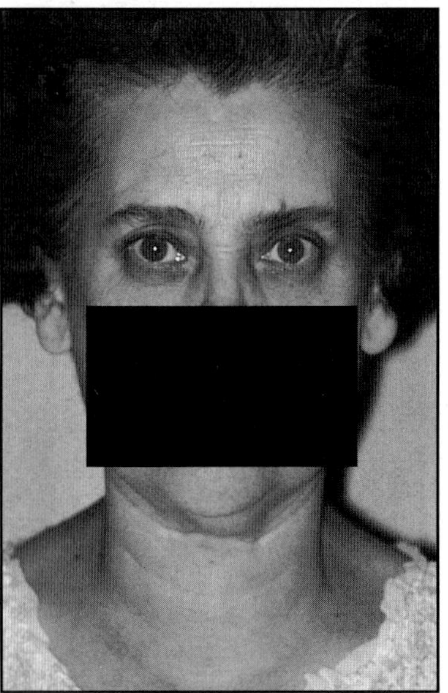

Note the eyes and the goitre of the patient; she attempted to treat herself by painting her neck with iodine.

EXAMINATION

On examination her pulse was 120 beats/min irregular, her jugular venous pressure was raised 5 cm and her blood pressure was 140/80 mmHg (mean). There was a split second heart sound and a soft systolic murmur. The lungs were clear. There was a small goitre and the liver edge was palpable. No abnormalities were detected on examining the eyes or nervous system.

Consider:

- **What is the likely diagnosis?**
- **What further clues to the underlying cause has the examination provided?**
- **What investigations should be performed?**

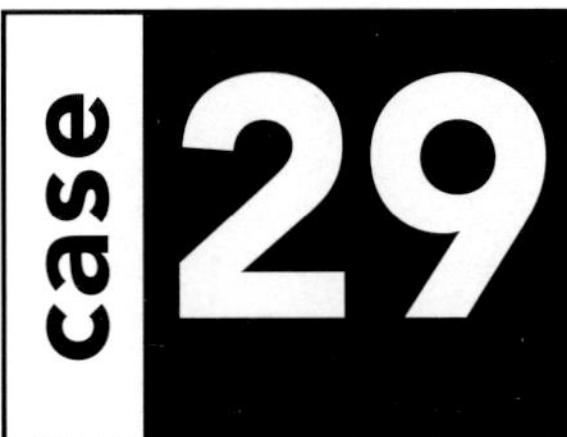

HISTORY

Paul Price, a 75-year-old man, was admitted via the emergency department to the ward. He lived alone and his neighbours, in the block of flats where he lived, had not seen him for a number of days and had contacted the emergency services. The police had to break down the door to gain access. The ambulance men reported that they found him lying in bed, fully conscious but reluctant to talk above monosyllables. There was an empty bottle of whiskey on the table and the room was filled with the smell of tobacco. On the journey to the hospital the ambulance personnel reported that he had been coughing and spitting into his handkerchief and that they had seen some blood mixed with his sputum.

He was equally reluctant to talk at first but after a time it was established that he had lived alone since his wife died 2 years previously. He admitted that he had not looked after himself well and had lost weight, although was uncertain by what amount. He had been sweating a lot recently. He had always had a 'smoker's cough' but recently this had been worse. He had been smoking 40 cigarettes a day but was reluctant to discuss his drinking habits. He revealed that this was the first time he had been in hospital since he was discharged from the army as medically unfit with a chest complaint in 1945.

Consider:
- **What are the two most important conditions to consider at this time?**
- **On examination, what would help to distinguish between these?**

EXAMINATION

The patient was somewhat reluctant to be examined but he certainly appeared to be wasted. His temperature was 37.5°C. His fingers were grossly stained with nicotine and appeared possibly clubbed. There were no spider naevi or other skin evidence of chronic liver disease. The chest examination showed some diminution of percussion note in the left upper chest anteriorly with poor breath sounds in the same area. The trachea appeared deviated to the left. In the abdomen, the liver appeared to be enlarged approximately 3 cm below the left costal margin and was smooth and nontender.

Consider:
- **How has the examination clarified the initial diagnoses?**

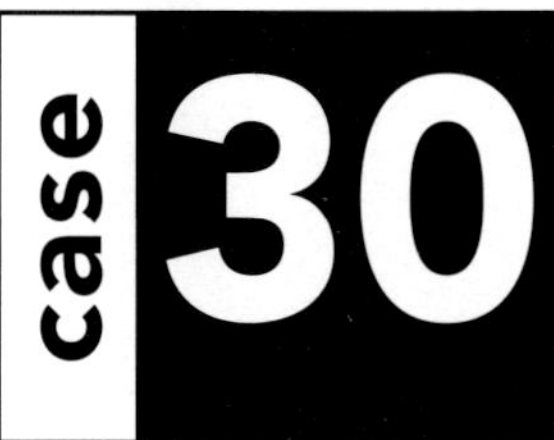

HISTORY

Scott Fleiss, a 20-year-old male student, was seen after an episode of fainting in the university gym. He collapsed after a round of circuit training and was apparently pulseless but recovered after a thump to the chest by a medical student. He refused immediate hospital admission and said he had felt well since.

Apart from the usual childhood illnesses, there was no significant medical history. His father died at the age of 70 years from cancer and his mother was alive and 50 years old. A step sister died suddenly at the age of 25 years but he did not know the details.

He had never previously had syncope but had recently noticed short bouts of rapid palpitation after rowing.

Consider:

- **What are the likely causes of syncope under these circumstances?**
- **Are there any further details that should be sought from the family history?**
- **Is there anyone else who could give useful information?**

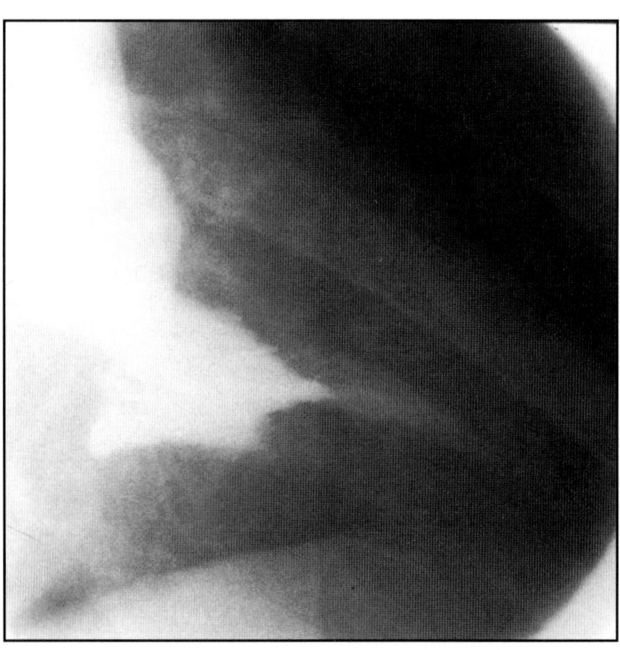

The patient's left ventricular cine angiogram.

EXAMINATION

On examination the patient was a fit, healthy-looking young man. His blood pressure was 110/70 mmHg, his pulse was 60 beats/min and his jugular venous pressure was not elevated. The cardiac apex was forceful and had a double character. It was also possible to see a double beat to the cardiac apex on inspecting the chest. There was a fourth heart sound and a soft ejection systolic murmur that got louder during a Valsalva manoeuvre. The carotid pulse felt jerky.

Consider:

- **What do the physical signs suggest?**
- **How can they be explained?**
- **What further tests need to be done?**

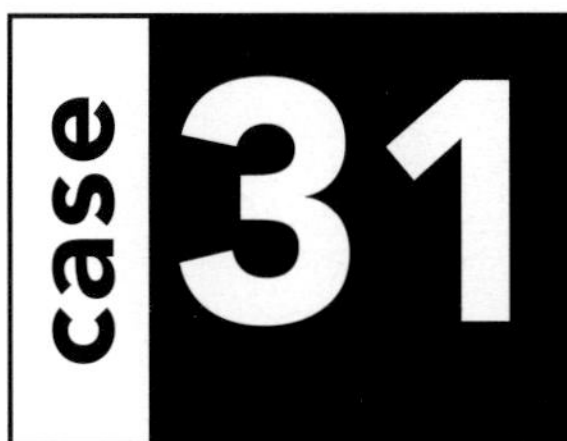

HISTORY

Richard O'Hearn, a 65-year-old man, had been referred by his general practitioner for a second opinion. The referring practitioner's letter stated that he believed the patient to be in heart failure, although he had not responded to treatment. The patient himself revealed that he had been getting more short of breath on exertion for the previous 2 months so that now he could only walk approximately 100 metres before he had to stop for a rest; he often had to stop when walking up a flight of stairs. There was little variation in his symptoms from day to day. He slept well on two pillows and there had been no ankle swelling. He had no chest pain or wheeze but he had had a long-standing morning cough with grey sputum.

He had smoked 20 cigarettes a day but had stopped approximately 5 years previously. He had spent all his adult life working in the construction industry as an electrician. He had never worked with asbestos. The only pet at home was his wife's budgerigar.

He confirmed that although his doctor's treatment made him pass a lot of water, it had not helped his breathlessness. He was on no other medication.

Consider:

- **What is the most likely causes of his breathlessness and why?**
- **What is the significance of the social factors in this history?**
- **What should be looked for on examination and why?**

EXAMINATION

The patient appeared breathless on getting undressed but otherwise seemed well. There might be some clubbing of the fingers but there was no cyanosis or ankle oedema. The cardiovascular system examination appeared normal; his pulse rate was 85 beats/min and his blood pressure was 135/90 mmHg. In the respiratory system examination, the trachea was central, the expansion of the chest appeared equal but reduced and the percussion note seemed slightly reduced at both lung bases. There were also marked crackles at both bases heard later in inspiration. The rest of the examination was normal.

Consider:

- **How has the examination helped clarify suspicions?**
- **What is the significance of the apparent dullness at both lung bases?**

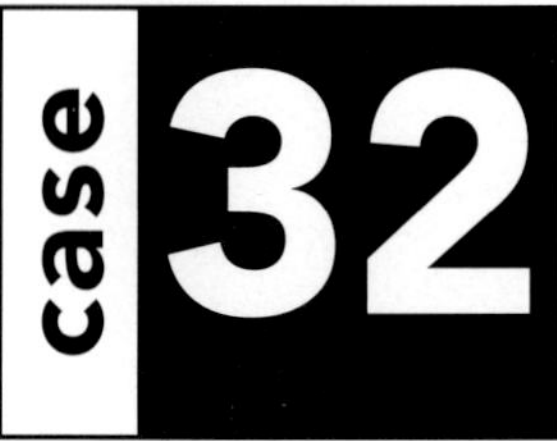

HISTORY

Rosalie Elliott, a 71-year-old retired woman, complained of weight loss. She said she had lost at least 15 kg over a 1-year period. During this time she had visited her doctor on a couple of occasions complaining of epigastric pains. These were intermittent and colicky in nature. She had noted that the pains seemed to be worse around meal times. This had led to a reduction in her appetite and she had reduced the size of her meals in an attempt to avoid the pain. A barium meal arranged at the start of her symptomatology had been reported as normal. She had become worried about her weight loss because all her friends had started to comment on how thin she was.

She had not noticed any change in her bowel habit. She did pass more urine recently. She had had a myocardial infarct when aged 66 years. She took a junior aspirin each day. The recently prescribed H_2 blocker had not helped her stomach pains. She was a nonsmoker and admitted to enjoying sherry in the afternoons with her friends.

Consider:
- **What are the most important causes of weight loss?**
- **Which organ is likely to be affected, causing her weight loss?**
- **What is the likely cause of her urinary frequency?**
- **Does the history indicate a possible predisposing factor?**

EXAMINATION

The patient was very thin, with evidence of cachexia. There was no lymphadenopathy or pallor. Abdominal examination showed moderate epigastric tenderness and an easily palpable aorta. This was not felt to be aneurysmal. No other masses were felt. Rectal examination revealed no masses and a pale stool. No blood was present. Breast examination did not detect any lumps. Cardiovascular and respiratory examination was entirely normal. The only finding on neurological examination was a concomitant squint that the patient said she was born with.

Consider:
- **How does the abdominal examination explain her weight loss?**
- **Why are her stools pale?**
- **What investigations would help support the clinical diagnosis?**

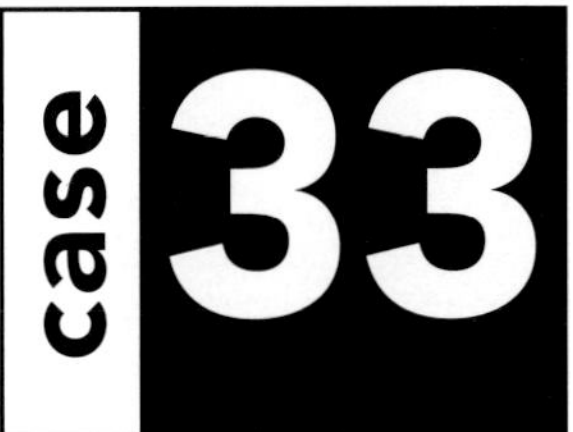

HISTORY

Jim O'Reilly, a 48-year-old bar manager, had been well previously although he had had a tendency to hypertension for some years. A year before, he had had an episode of acute pain in the right ankle. The pain had been associated with redness and swelling. He had visited his general practitioner who had diagnosed arthritis and prescribed the nonsteriodal anti-inflammatory drug, naproxen. The pain and swelling had subsided over a few days and no further action had been taken.

He presented to Casualty a year later at 9 a.m. He had woken at 3 a.m. with intense pain in his right big toe which had, if anything, increased in severity. He had sweated profusely and felt shivery. The area around the big toe had become exquisitely tender, so that he had had to remove the bed clothes. He had been unable to get back to sleep and because it was the weekend, had decided to come to casualty.

His health had otherwise been satisfactory. The casualty officer noted that the patient's general practitioner had started bendrofluazide 2 weeks previously because of an elevated blood pressure reading. The patient had been a nonsmoker for 3 years but regularly consumed 4 pints of beer a day (56 units a week).

Consider:
- **What is the likely diagnosis?**
- **Is the patient's lifestyle likely to be relevant?**
- **Is the prescription of a diuretic 2 weeks before significant?**

EXAMINATION

The patient was acutely distressed and clearly in severe pain. His blood pressure was 150/110 mmHg, his pulse was 110 beats/min and he was in sinus rhythm. He was obese (92 kg). He had a low grade fever (37.5°C). The general systems examination was normal. Abnormalities were confined to the right foot; the whole foot and ankle were swollen. There was marked redness over the metatarsophalangeal joint of the big toe that extended on to the dorsum of the foot. The joint was exquisitely tender and the patient would hardly allow the examination.

The casualty officer organised a radiograph of the foot and ankle. This showed no specific abnormality. A peripheral blood film showed a white cell count of 12 000/mm^3 with 85% being polymorphonuclear leukocytes. He arranged a further blood test and prescribed indomethacin in a dose of 50 mg four times daily. The patient returned 48 h later. By then there had been a dramatic improvement with lessening of pain and swelling. The joint was less red and far less tender. The indomethacin was continued for a further week in a reducing dose.

Consider:
- **What blood test was ordered?**
- **What alternative method is available for establishing the diagnosis?**
- **What long-term management can be offered?**

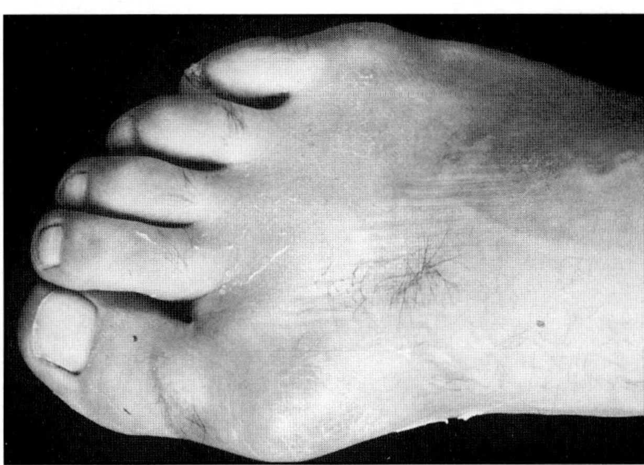

The patient's right foot.

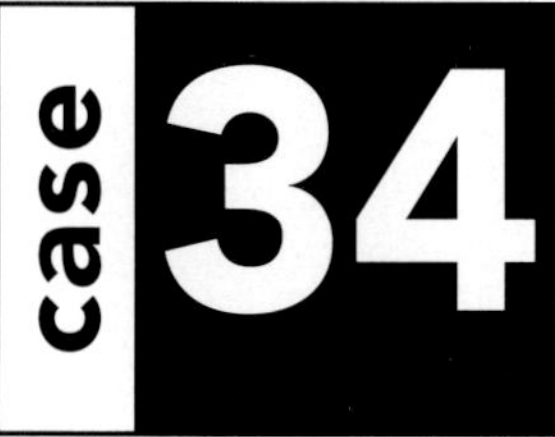

HISTORY

Madurhi Kaur, a 65-year-old female Asian immigrant, presented to her family doctor with abdominal discomfort and increasing abdominal distension of 3 weeks' duration. In addition, she had lost 5 kg in weight over the preceding 4 weeks.

She also complained of increasing difficulty with her breathing for the past fortnight. This was particularly apparent on lying down but improved on standing.

She had a medical history of ischaemic heart disease with an inferior myocardial infarction 2 years previously for which she was taking aspirin and atenolol. She had never smoked and was a teetotaller. There was also no relevant family history.

Consider:
- **What are the causes of abdominal distention?**
- **Why might her breathing be affected?**

EXAMINATION

The patient appeared comfortable at rest without any evidence of dyspnoea. Her temperature was 36.8°C. She was, however, cachectic with prominent cheek bones and drawing of the cheeks. There was no palmar erythema, spider naevi or jaundice.

Her pulse was 60 beats/min regular with a normal character. The first and second heart sounds were normal. Her jugular venous pressure was not elevated and her blood pressure was 130/80 mmHg. There was no peripheral oedema. Her chest was clear and breath sounds were vesicular.

Abdominal examination revealed a generalised symmetrically distended tense abdomen with shifting dullness on percussion of the flanks. There were no palpable masses. Rectal examination did not reveal any abnormality. The neurological examination was normal.

Consider:
- **What is the likely cause of the shifting dullness?**
- **What negative physical sign helps refine the differential diagnosis?**
- **What test would help make a definitive diagnosis?**

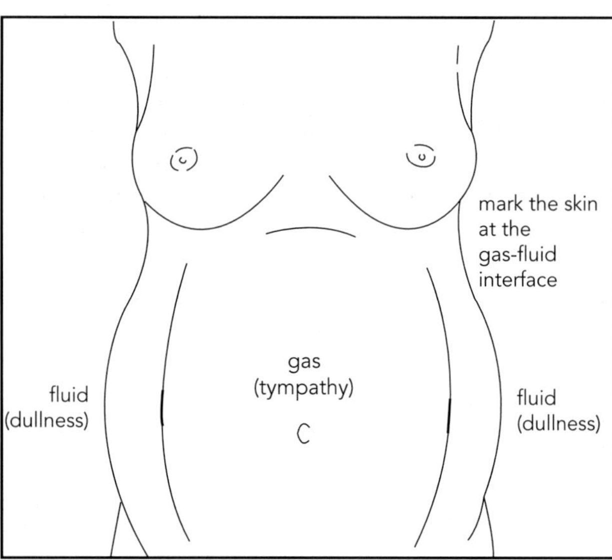

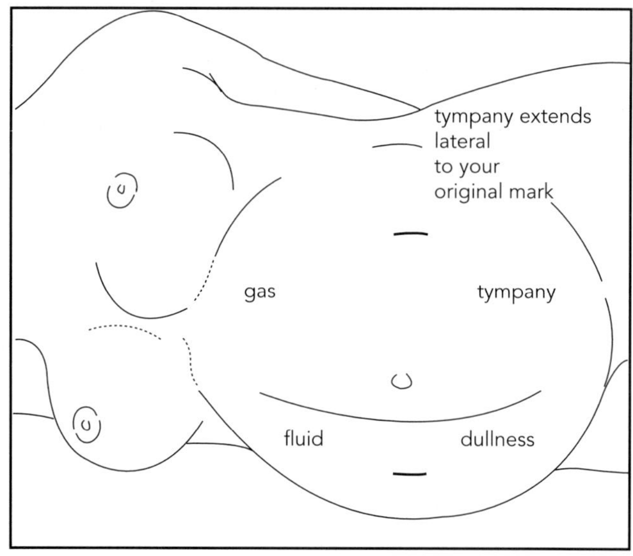

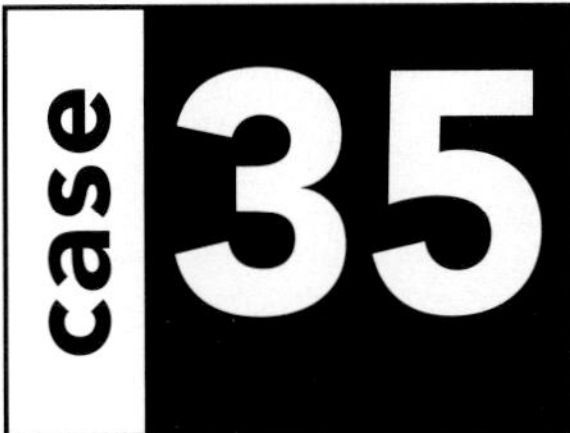

HISTORY

Kwan Ju Lee, a 54-year-old man, had had a fairly chequered medical history, with recurrent pneumothoraces, a perforated appendix, a protracted whiplash injury after a road traffic accident and subsequent chronic neck pain. The neck pain had been treated by various means, including physiotherapy, manipulation and, most recently, acupuncture. The exact basis for the pain remained uncertain because routine cervical spine radiographs had shown little. The patient had become severely disgruntled by the problem and was taking medico-legal action.

For approximately a year the patient had noticed a swelling in his right groin that had gradually increased in size. The swelling varied and he noticed it became more prominent when coughing. His doctor had told him of the diagnosis (an inguinal hernia) but the patient refused referral for a surgical opinion. Twenty-four hours before his eventual admission he had had a bout of violent coughing (he was a heavy smoker), as he did, the pain in his groin became intense. When he inspected the hernia, he found it had increased in size and appeared much less compressible than normal. Over the next few hours the pain persisted and he developed increasing colicky abdominal pain. He was admitted.

On examination he was distressed. He had an irreducible right inguinal hernia which was tender. He vomited during the examination. The rest of his general and neurological examination was normal. He underwent laparotomy. There was an incarcerated inguinal hernia. It was felt that a short segment of the bowel was no longer viable and 6 cm were excised with an end to end anastomosis. He had a stormy postoperative course and was on intravenous fluids and antibiotics for several days.

On the seventh postoperative day, as the drip was being taken down from his right arm, he commented to the nursing staff that he had some numbness in his right little finger and that his right hand felt slightly weak and clumsy. A doctor came to assess the problem.

Consider:

- **Is the problem likely to be in the central or peripheral nervous system?**
- **How will the distribution of any sensory or motor deficit in the left arm aid diagnosis?**

EXAMINATION

The neurological abnormalities were confined to the right arm. There was no wasting or fasciculation and no change in the reflexes. Muscle tone was normal, as was co-ordination. There was consistent weakness in the interossei (4/5) together with weakness of a similar degree in abductor digiti minimi and adductor pollicis. Abductor pollicis brevis, on the other hand, appeared normal. The long flexors of the fingers appeared intact, as did both flexor carpi ulnaris and flexor carpi radialis. Tinel's sign was negative at the elbow. He was not a good sensory witness but appeared to have reduced cutaneous sensation on the little finger and the ulnar border of the hand. The findings in the ring finger were inconsistent.

Consider:

- **Has the examination confirmed the nature of the problem?**
- **To where can the problem be localised?**
- **Why has this happened?**

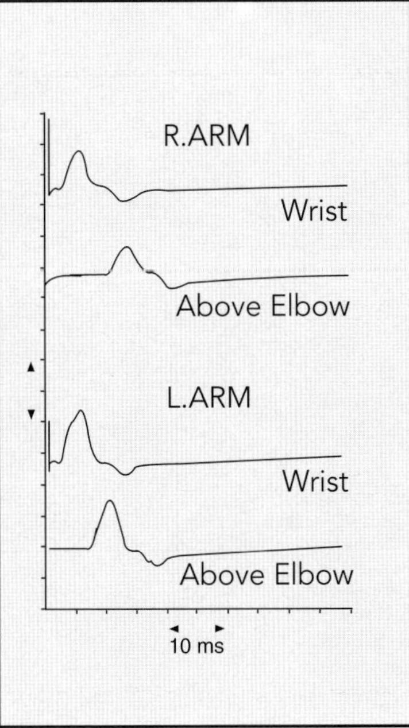

This figure compares the potentials from abductor digiti minimi in the right and left arms obtained by stimulating the ulnar nerve at the wrist and above the elbow.

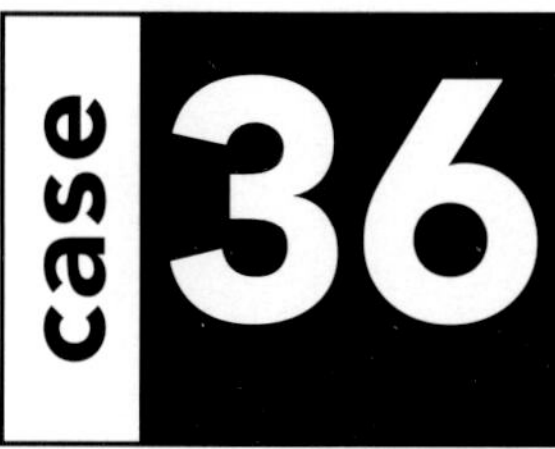

HISTORY

Lee Chang, a six-and-a-half-year-old boy, was seen in the paediatric clinic with a 10-day history of coughing. His parents reported that he was sleeping poorly because of paroxysms of coughing that were particularly bad at night. He was also coughing during the day, particularly on exertion.

The boy had been seen previously with eczema and both his parents were moderately heavy smokers.

Consider:
- **What are the most important differential diagnoses?**
- **What history and examination findings are of interest?**

EXAMINATION

The boy looked tired. His height and weight followed the 25th centile. He had no respiratory distress at rest. He was pink and well perfused. His chest shape was normal. His peak expiratory flow rate was 105 l/min (<fifth centile for height). The rest of the examination was uninformative.

Consider:
- **Has the examination confirmed the initial differential diagnosis?**
- **What is the management plan**
- **Should any other questions be asked?**

There was a family history of atopy and smoking. Asthma may present as cough in the absence of wheeze. His peak expiratory flow rate was less than the mean for his height. A therapeutic trial of asthma treatment with inhaled β_2 agonists and a short course of oral steroids with an asthma diary with daily home peak flow measurements was arranged.

Three days later on review the boy was no better. His parents reported that doing the peak expiratory flow measurements induced paroxysms of coughing and the inhaled salbutamol (via spacer) was no help. A peak flow measurement in theclinic induced a spasm of coughing. After several coughs the boy inhaled noisily and continued to cough with his tongue protruding. He became mildly cyanosed before the paroxysm finished.

It is discovered that the boy's immunisation history is incomplete; the pertussis component was omitted at the mother's insistence. His mother says the cough has been as dramatic as the episode witnessed. He had not coughed before this illness.

A pernasal swab was sent and a full blood count showed the following results:

Haemoglobin	**11.9 g/dl**
White blood cell count	**21 x 10^9/l (2.4 neutrophils, 18.3 lymphocytes)**
Platelets	**319 x 10^{12} /l**

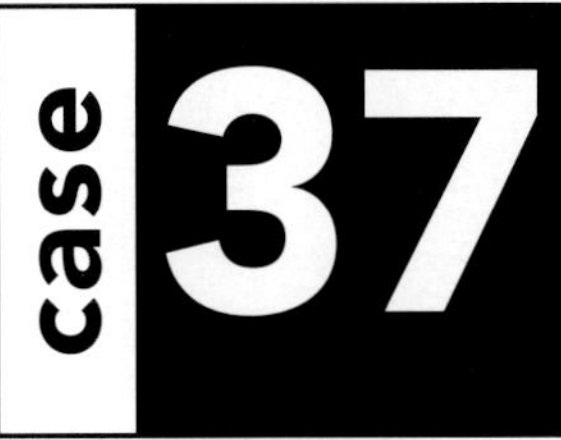

HISTORY

George Becker, a 62-year-old man, had a hoarse voice for 4 weeks. The hoarseness was constant and his voice quality was deteriorating. He had no pain or difficulty in swallowing. He had no earache. His appetite was good and he had not lost weight.

He worked as a marketing consultant and had to use his voice daily giving lectures, presentations and so on. He smoked 20 cigarettes a day and drank 15 units of alcohol a week.

He had had no other illnesses relevant to his upper aerodigestive tract. He had had what he called a 'smoker's cough' for many years but had never coughed up any blood.

Consider:
- **What diagnosis must be most likely and why?**
- **Is the problem related to excessive voice usage or smoking?**
- **What examinations should be carried out?**

EXAMINATION

The patient appeared clinically well and was not short of breath. The oral cavity revealed staining of his teeth from long-term cigarette smoking and his tongue was furred. His tonsils were small and the buccal mucosa showed no evidence of any focal disease.

His postnasal space, hypopharynx and larynx were examined by indirect methods using laryngeal and postnasal mirrors. A direct examination was then performed using a flexible nasendoscope. A small exophytic lesion was found arising from the left vocal fold. There was normal movement of the vocal folds.

Palpation of the neck revealed no thyromegaly or lymphadenopathy.

Consider:
- **Are there any predisposing factors in the history?**
- **Has the examination given the diagnosis?**
- **Are any other investigations necessary?**

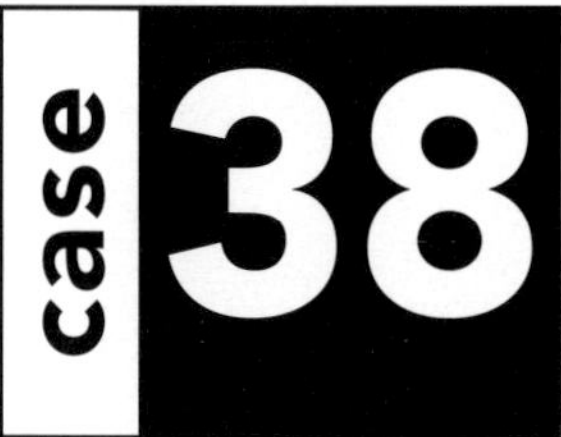

HISTORY

Bob Bacchus, a 60-year-old man, was seen because of chest pain on exertion. He was well until a month ago, since then he had noticed chest pain on walking progressively shorter distances. The pain was retrosternal and radiated to the jaw and it was accompanied by an ache in the left arm; it was worse when he exercised after a meal or outside in the cold. For the past 2 days he had had a similar pain at rest. He smoked 20 cigarettes a day. His father died from a heart attack aged 50 years.

Consider:
- **What is the most likely diagnosis?**
- **What could account for the various factors that precipitate the pain?**
- **What could be made of the progressive nature of his symptoms?**

EXAMINATION

Shortly after climbing on to the examination couch, the patient complained of further pain which persisted and became severe. He started sweating, looked pale and his skin felt cold and clammy. His pulse was 90 beats/min with frequent extra beats and his blood pressure was 110/90 mmHg.

Consider:
- **What could be happening?**
- **What could cause the physical signs?**
- **What should be done?**

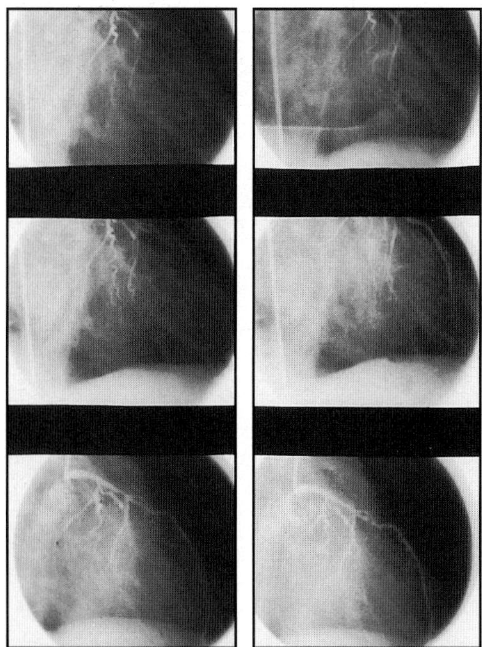

The patient's coronary angiogram.

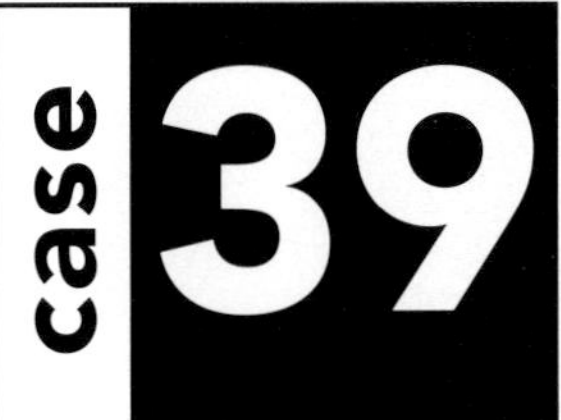

HISTORY

Barbara Bustamente, a 65-year-old woman, had had a myocardial infarct 3 years previously. She was known to be hypertensive and had developed noninsulin-dependent diabetes mellitus the previous summer. Two months before her admission she had complained to her husband of a short-lived episode of clumsiness of the right hand but had not sought medical advice. On the day of her admission she had suddenly become unable to speak while on the telephone to her daughter. Almost immediately she developed weakness of the right arm and leg and had difficulty remaining standing. She was admitted to hospital. Her husband indicated that she was right handed. There was no relevant family history.

Consider:

- **What may be the significance of the event 2 months before?**
- **Why is the history of her handedness important?**
- **What underlying pathology is suspected?**

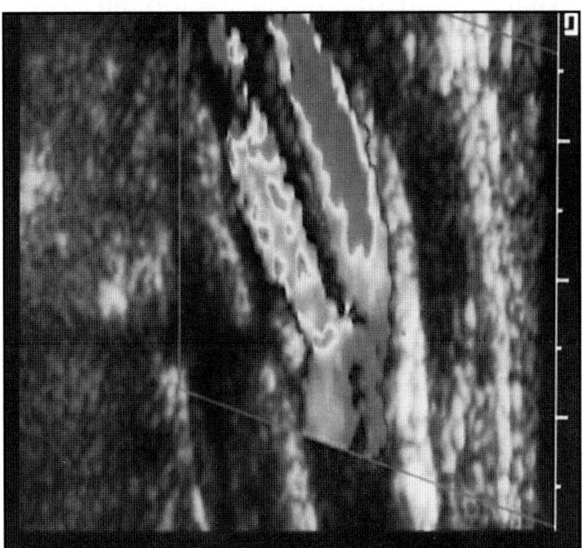

A Doppler study of the patient's left carotid bifurcation.

EXAMINATION

On examination the patient was alert. She appeared to understand fully and could carry out complex instructions providing she was not required to use her right side. Her spontaneous speech was severely reduced and lacking in grammatical content; often her responses were reduced to single words. Her visual fields were full. The cranial nerve examination was normal, except for a right upper motor neuron facial weakness. She had a moderate (grade 4/5) right-sided pyramidal weakness. Tone was normal, reflexes symmetrical but the right plantar response was weakly extensor. Her sensation appeared intact. Co-ordination on the right side was difficult to assess but appeared normal on the left.

The general systems' examination was fairly unremarkable in that her blood pressure was normal (148/90 mmHg) and she was in sinus rhythm and had normal peripheral pulses. There was a suggestion of bruits bilaterally over the carotid bifurcations.

She began to improve rapidly, so that within 48 h she was able to walk unassisted and was able to hold objects fairly well in her right hand. By then her speech was better, although reduced in content. She was able to indicate she had a substantial, predominantly left-sided headache.

Consider:

- **What type of speech disorder is this?**
- **How might fundoscopy provide a clue to the mechanism of these events?**
- **What assessment of her arterial tree might provide valuable data about the mechanism of her stroke?**
- **What therapeutic options will be influenced by the findings of this investigation?**

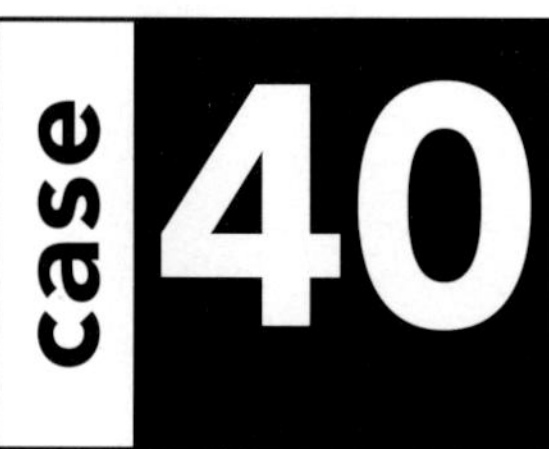

HISTORY

John Knight, a 65-year-old married businessman, presented to casualty after noting black, offensive stools for the previous 24 h. He also complained of upper abdominal pain, partly relieved with ingestion of yoghurt. There was no nausea or vomiting and his appetite remained unchanged. He had not noticed weight loss or a change in his bowel habit.

The patient smoked a pipe. Daily business lunches and a few night caps resulted in a weekly alcohol intake of up to 80 units.

He had no medical history or family history of note. He was taking no regular medication at the time of presentation but did take ibuprofen quite often for headaches.

Consider:
- **Where does melena stool arise from?**
- **What predisposing factors are evident from the history?**
- **Which is the most likely cause of melena without vomiting blood?**

EXAMINATION

The patient appeared to be unwell. He was pale and sweaty. On inspection of his hands there was palmar erythema but no flapping tremor was noted. There was a hint of jaundice and a few spider naevi were noted on his arms and chest wall.

His pulse was 100 beats/min regular and of small volume. His blood pressure was 110/70 mmHg supine, dropping to 90/60 mmHg in the upright position. His jugular venous pressure was not visible. His first and second heart sounds and respiratory examination were normal with vesicular breath sounds.

Abdominal examination revealed a tender liver with the edge palpable 6 cm below the costal margin. There was no shifting dullness but the spleen was palpable 1 cm below the left costal margin. There was dullness to percussion in the ninth intercostal space, anterior to the axillary line. Rectal examination revealed melena stool.

The neurological examination was normal.

Consider:
- **What is the likely diagnosis?**
- **What investigation would confirm the diagnosis?**

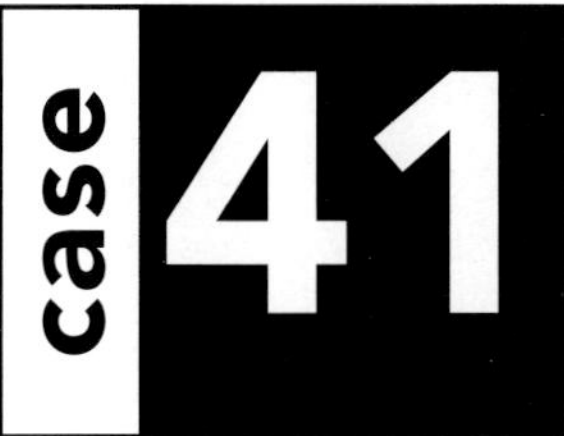

HISTORY

Marshall Martin, a 50-year-old man, had had little in the way of medical problems until his wife's death 3 years previously. He lived alone, having never had children. He worked in the computer industry and frequently took trips abroad. Although he had never smoked, he had always drunk alcohol regularly, perhaps averaging 30 units a week in the past. At a company medical a year before, his gamma glutamyl transferase level had been slightly elevated and the company doctor had advised him to reduce his intake. Soon afterwards he fractured his leg in a skiing accident and had to be off work for a month. On his return to work, his colleagues noticed that his work had become a little less reliable and that he periodically arrived late in the mornings. He appeared dispirited by his failure to achieve promotion to a post he had particularly coveted and one that would have dramatically reduced his travel commitment. He began to have bouts of unexplained vomiting which he told his colleagues were attributable to a peptic ulcer. It was noticeable that his appetite had diminished and that he was losing weight. Over a 3-week period, his work attendance became increasingly erratic. During this time, his walking appeared less stable and he complained of numbness in his feet. At the end of this period, he was found in bed at home on a Monday morning by his domestic cleaner. He appeared confused and unwell and she called for an ambulance to take him to hospital.

Only a limited history was possible from the patient. He had clearly lost weight and appeared dehydrated. He was uncertain of the date and of his whereabouts. He suggested that he had been at work regularly and even detailed a major business deal that he had recently completed in Frankfurt. His employers subsequently indicated that he had not travelled to Germany for the past year. He indicated that his alcohol intake had been unchanged.

Consider:
- **What do the patient's limb symptoms suggest?**
- **What is the patient's mental state?**
- **What is the working diagnosis?**

EXAMINATION

On examination his short-term memory was poor and erratic. At the time, he produced details that appeared unlikely to be correct from the known history. His general systems examination revealed a tender liver, approximately 5 cm below the costal margin. He had normal fundi but there was evidence of bilateral sixth nerve palsies with vertical nystagmus on upward gaze. His tongue and limbs were tremulous. He appeared to have bilateral upper and lower limb ataxia. He refused to get out of bed. Power was probably intact and tone normal. The reflexes were present apart from absent ankle jerks. The plantars were equivocal. Sensory testing was difficult but pin prick, at least, appeared blunted in the feet.

Consider:
- **What conclusions can be drawn from the physical findings?**
- **What simple blood tests would be helpful in confirming your suspicions?**
- **What might computerised tomography or magnetic resonance imaging of the head show?**
- **What treatment should be started?**
- **What is the likely outcome?**

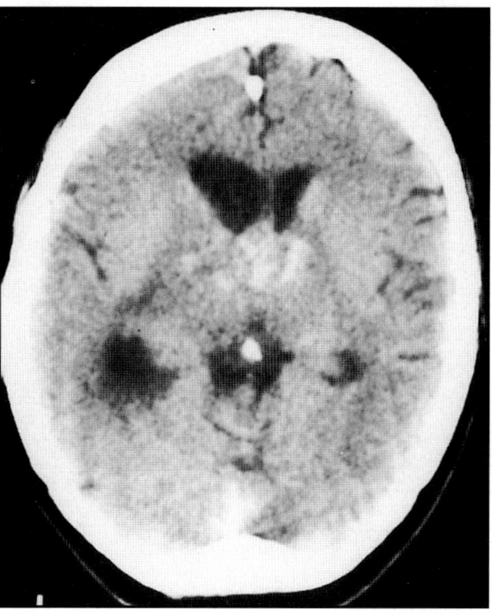

The patient's CT scan.

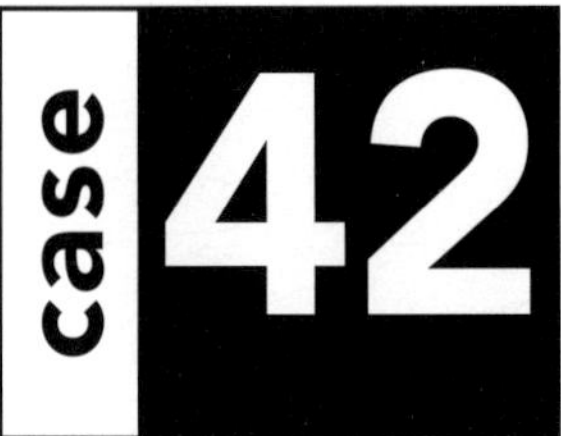

HISTORY

Rosa Fernandez, a 45-year-old woman, was referred on account of palpitations. She had had occasional palpitations in the past but her symptoms had become worse over the past 3 months. The palpitation was most troublesome at the end of the day or when she relaxed after work; she occasionally woke up with it. She described a feeling as though her heart momentarily stopped, followed by a thump. She did not have palpitation during exercise.

A few months ago she was found to have mildly high blood pressure and was started on bendrofluazide 5 mg daily. Her general practitioner had tried putting her on atenolol but this did not relieve the symptoms.

Consider:
- **Does the history give any clues to the likely cause of the palpitation?**
- **Are these symptoms likely to be caused by anxiety?**
- **Is the drug history of any relevance?**

EXAMINATION

The patient looked fit and well. Her pulse was 70 beats/min regular but with the frequent ectopic beats. Her cardiac apex was normal, there was a soft mid to late systolic murmur and her jugular venous pressure was not raised. Her blood pressure was 150/90 mmHg.

Consider:
- **Is there any evidence of cardiac enlargement?**
- **Is there any evidence of a valve defect?**
- **Why is this important?**

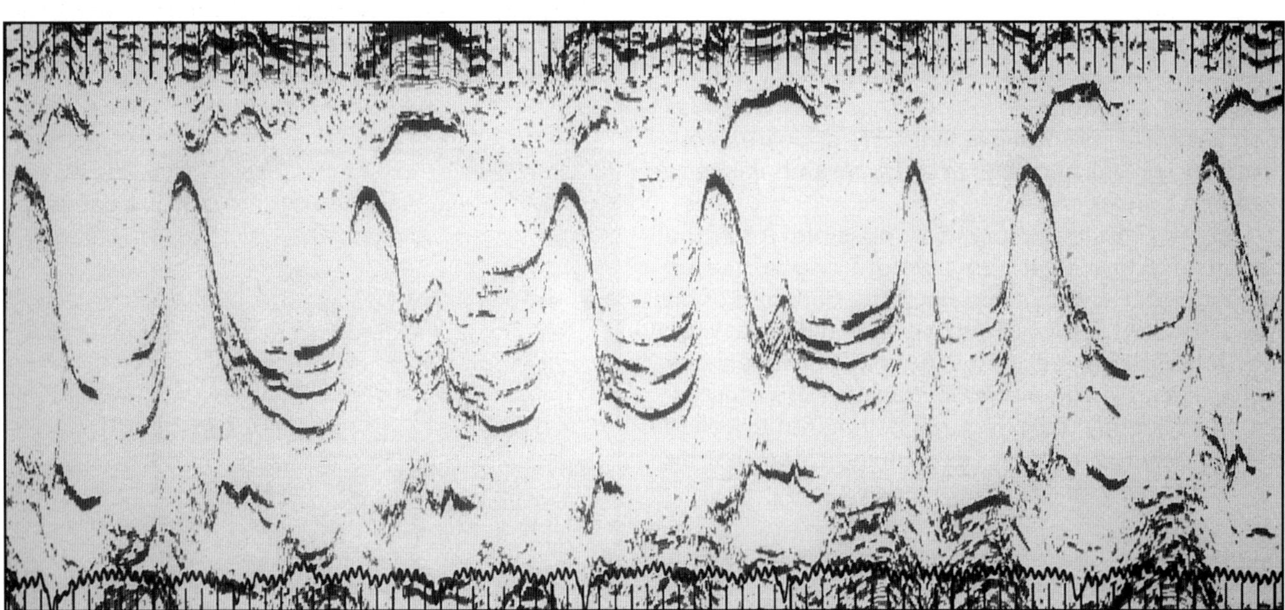

The patient's echocardiogram.

case 43

HISTORY

Luigi Gianetto, a 70-year-old man, was retired and had been in poor health for some years. He had been found to be hypertensive at the time of a myocardial infarct 8 years before. Control of his blood pressure had been poor, partly because of poor compliance with medication, which the patient freely admitted. Despite frequent rejoinders, he had continued to smoke 20 cigarettes a day. His alcohol consumption was modest. Four years before he had been investigated for possible polycythaemia but in the end the diagnosis could not be sustained and he had not received treatment.

On the day of admission he had appeared well in the morning but shortly after lunch he suddenly developed an intense headache over the left occipital region. At the same time he almost lost his balance and realised that he was staggering to the left. When reaching out with his left hand to support himself, he found that the hand appeared clumsy. He remained fully alert. He had an ill-defined sense of vertigo and vomited once. He had no other neurological complaints. His angina, which had persisted on and off since his infarct, had been rather worse recently. Besides his blood pressure and angina medication, he was on low-dose aspirin (75 mg/day).

Consider:
- **Where would you place this patient's stroke?**
- **What is the likely pathology?**

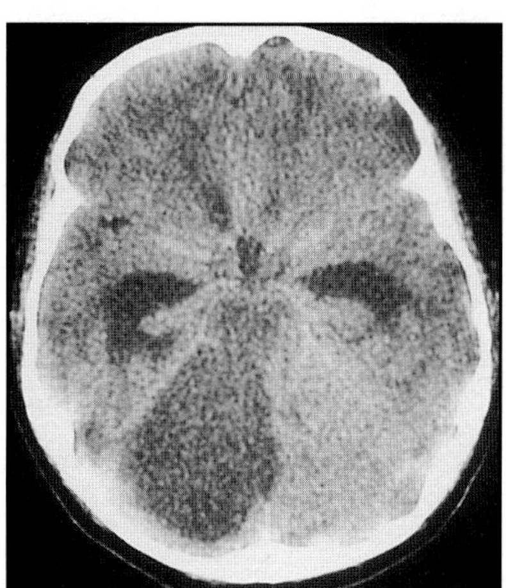

The repeat CT scan performed four days after the onset of disability.

EXAMINATION

On examination he was fully alert. His blood pressure was 190/110 mmHg and he was in sinus rhythm. The peripheral pulses were intact. His heart appeared slightly enlarged with a displaced apex and his aortic second sound was accentuated. He appeared rather plethoric and was overweight. His fundi showed arteriovenous crossing changes. There was a first degree jerk nystagmus to the left. The rest of the cranial nerve examination was normal. His left hand was clumsy with a tendency to past point. The left heel–knee–shin test was ataxic. Right-sided co-ordination was satisfactory. Limb power and tone appeared normal. The reflexes were symmetrical; the left plantar was equivocal, the right plantar was flexor. His sensation was normal. He was reluctant to get out of bed and if he did so, he immediately staggered to the left.

The admitting physician ordered an urgent computerised tomography scan which was performed within 8 h of the onset of his symptoms. The scan was normal. The physician diagnosed some form of brainstem stroke and advised bed rest. Within 72 h the patient's condition had substantially deteriorated. He was now very drowsy and physical examination proved difficult. There appeared to be a slight impairment of abduction of the left eye and the left nasolabial fold seemed flattened. His palate elevated poorly and because of choking he could no longer tolerate oral fluids. The limb signs remained but both plantars were now extensor.

Consider:
- **Has the examination confirmed the site of the pathology?**
- **What investigation would be most helpful?**
- **Why do you think the patient's condition has deteriorated and how would you manage the problem?**

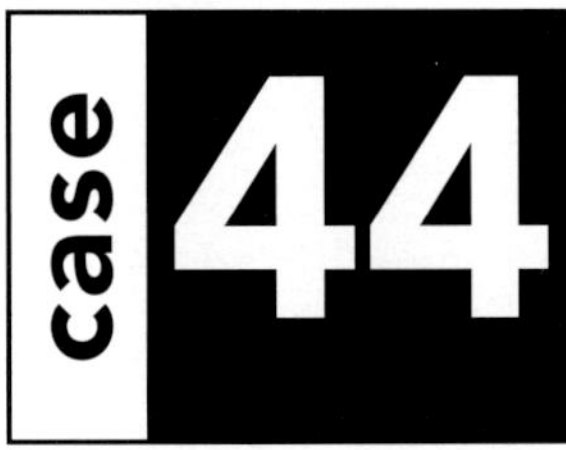

HISTORY

Carrie Blanca, an 8-month-old girl, was referred by the Accident and Emergency staff. She had presented with a unilateral left parietal swelling and skull radiographs confirmed a left parietal skull fracture.

The referring doctor was anxious because there had been no recent history of injury. Her mother was vague about this but she mentioned that her husband said that the infant had rolled off the parents' bed while he was changing a nappy, 3 days previously. The baby appeared well after this minor incident.

Consider:
- **What is the differential diagnoses?**
- **What history and examination findings are of interest?**
- **Do other professional agencies need to be involved?**

A more complete history was taken. The pregnancy and delivery were normal and the birth weight was 3.7 kg. The baby had been breast fed from birth, with the introduction of solids at 4 months of age. Her development had been normal so far; she had smiled at 4 weeks, sat unsupported at 6 months and could roll over but was not yet crawling. She had been fully immunised to date. She had a 22-month-old brother who was well. The parents were not married but they lived together. The father worked as a bus driver and the mother stopped working as a secretary when their first child was born.

The recent history was obtained from both parents; during the weekend, 3 days previously, the mother was out shopping with the 22-month-old brother. The father was caring for the baby and was changing her nappy on the parental bed. Half way through the changing the phone rang and the father went to answer it. His conversation was protracted and he had walked to another room to find his wallet while talking. After a period of approximatley 3–4 min, the father rushed back to the bedroom when he heard a thud and the baby wailing at the top of her voice.

The father picked her up off the carpeted floor (concrete under the underlay) and cuddled her for 10 min. She stopped crying after aaproximately 5 min and began to slowly cheer up. She did not vomit nor did she ever appear to lose consciousness. Later when the mother had returned, she played and fed normally. Two days before admission, the mother noticed a swelling on the left side of the baby's head. She made an appointment to see the family's general practitioner. This doctor referred them immediately to the Accident and Emergency department.

EXAMINATION

She appeared a happy infant with a firm tender swelling over the left parietal boss. Her head circumference was 47.3 cm (>97th centile) and her weight was 9.1 kg (<90th centile). Her pulse and blood pressure were normal. There were no focal neurological signs and her pupils were equal and reactive. There was no other bruising and she appeared well cared for.

Consider:
- **Has the further history and examination confirmed the initial differential diagnosis?**
- **What is the management plan?**

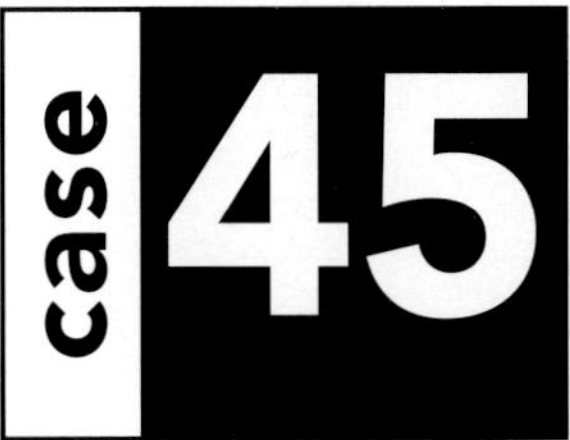

HISTORY

Lynda Matthews, a 35-year-old-woman, was referred to the clinic with recurrent episodes of shortness of breath. She had had a history of 'asthma' for a number of years consisting of episodes of variable wheezy breathlessness associated with a nonproductive cough. For the past year these episodes had been more severe and lasted longer and she had been increasingly unable to do her normal activities and had lost several weeks from work. Some episodes had been associated with 'dizziness' and light-headedness. She had continued her normal inhaled medication which sometimes gave her relief, although not as consistently as before. Some episodes were associated with pain along the left lower chest anteriorly which was also made worse on deep breathing. Many of the episodes were associated with exertion but some occurred at rest. She was waking up repeatedly at night with wheeze and shortness of breath. She had never smoked.

Consider:

- **What are the three conditions that should be considered at this time and why?**
- **What should be particularly looked for on examination to decide between these?**

EXAMINATION

The patient looked well although a little anxious. Her pulse was 84 beats/min and her blood pressure was 110/85 mmHg. The heart sounds were normal and there were no murmurs. In the respiratory system, the percussion note was normal but, on auscultation, there were a few scattered wheezes. On palpation there was some tenderness along the left costal margin that reproduced the pain. Her abdomen was normal. There was no tenderness or swelling of the legs. When the patient took 20 deep breaths, there were no additional symptoms.

Consider:

- **How has the examination clarified the initial diagnoses?**

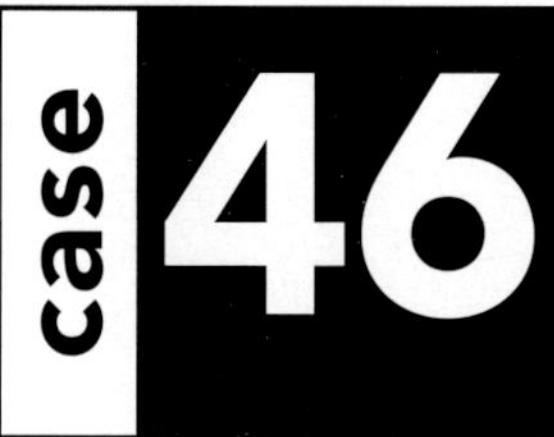

HISTORY

Alan Eldred, a 47-year-old married bar manager, presented to his family doctor complaining of upper abdominal discomfort. The discomfort was worse during periods of hunger and was relieved by the ingestion of milk. The pain was also relieved to some degree by simple antacids bought from a pharmacy. It was not relieved by posture. The episodes of upper abdominal pain had been occurring on an intermittent basis over the past 4 months and at times disturbed the patient from his sleep at night. He had noticed the pain radiating to the right of the abdomen and through to the back at times and he became nauseated during the episodes of pain. There had been no vomiting. His appetite had not been affected nor had he lost any weight. In the past he had not suffered from heartburn, odynophagia or dysphagia. He did not complain of abdominal bloating and his bowel habit had not changed.

He had had no medical or family history and, other than antacids, was on no regular medication. He smoked 20 cigarettes a day and he denied excessive drinking, although he agreed he was sociable.

Consider:
- **Which organs may cause food-related pain?**
- **What is the differential diagnosis?**
- **What aspect of the history suggests that the pain is organic rather than functional?**
- **How is the radiation of the pain helpful in determining which organ is affected?**

EXAMINATION

Examination revealed a well-nourished and hydrated man. There was no jaundice, pallor or lymphadenopathy.

The cardiovascular system examination revealed a normal first and second heart sound and respiratory examination revealed vesicular breath sounds. The neurological examination was normal.

On examination of the abdomen there was mild tenderness in the epigastric region but Murphy's sign was negative. There was no clinical enlargement of the liver, spleen or kidneys or evidence of any free fluid in the abdomen. The bowel sounds were normal and there were no abdominal bruits. The rectal examination was normal.

Consider:
- **What is the relevance of a negative Murphy's sign?**
- **What investigation would help make a firm diagnosis?**

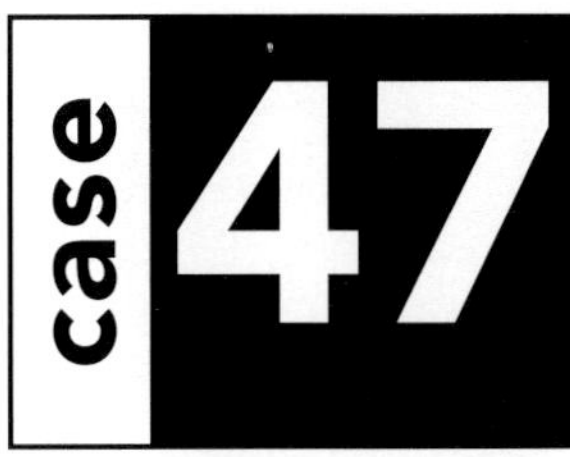

HISTORY

Chuck Lukach, a 30-year-old male weight-lifter, had been in excellent health in the past. He was single. He had always refused to use illicit drugs in aiding his career (they had frequently been available) and despite this had represented his country at the Olympic Games. Like many of his fellow athletes, his back could trouble him from time to time and he always wore a support when lifting, even though he appreciated that its value was limited.

He was competing in his national championships and had already won his title but decided to attempt a national record with his last lift. He expected to retire from the sport and concentrate on his other love, sheep farming. He realised that the weight was at the limit of his capacity. As he lifted the final phase, he developed an intense low back pain. Somehow he sustained the lift for the statutory period but then had to immediately drop the weight, narrowly escaping injury. The pain persisted and appeared to extend to his buttocks bilaterally. He insisted on returning to his hotel room to rest rather than seeking immediate medical attention. Already he was aware of an ill-defined numbness in the posterior thighs. He took several aspirins and went to bed.

On waking the pain was still present and the numbness, if anything, more intense. He struggled out of bed but realised that his feet were weak and he had difficulty getting to the toilet. His bladder felt somewhat full and he decided to sit on the toilet to micturate. He realized that his buttocks were numb and, to his horror, found he could not pass urine. He rang for an ambulance and was admitted to hospital. He had no other neurological complaints and, apart from an occasional tendency to wheeze (for which he tried to avoid taking medication because of his concerns about drug testing), he was well.

Consider:

- **Where is the pathological process likely to be situated?**
- **What neurological structure has been disturbed?**

EXAMINATION

On neurological examination his cranial nerves and upper limbs were normal. He was tender over the lumbosacral junction. Straight leg raising was limited to 20° bilaterally, evoking posterior thigh pain on either side. Femoral stretch was negative. He had weakness of planter flexion, knee flexion and hip extension bilaterally. The knee jerks were brisk and the ankle jerks absent. The plantars were weakly flexor. Tone was normal and co-ordination intact. He had blunting of cutaneous sensation over the posterior thighs extending to the perianal region bilaterally. His anal sphincter tone was reduced. His bladder was palpable to the umbilicus. A general systems examination was satisfactory.

Consider:

- **What segments are affected on the basis of the motor assessment?**
- **What segments are affected on the basis of the sensory assessment?**
- **What investigation would be most helpful?**
- **How would you manage this problem?**

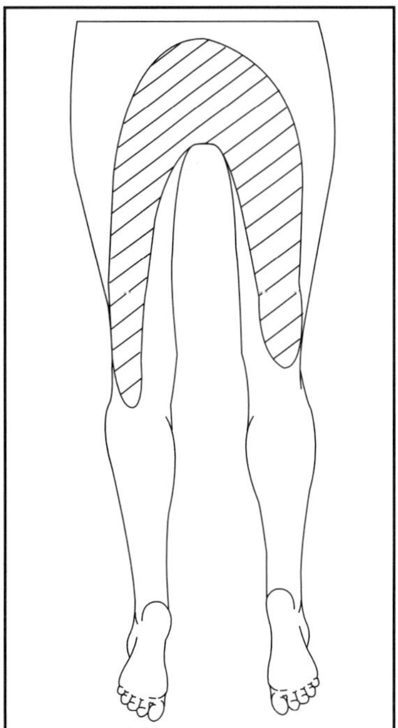

The distribution of the cutaneous sensory loss.

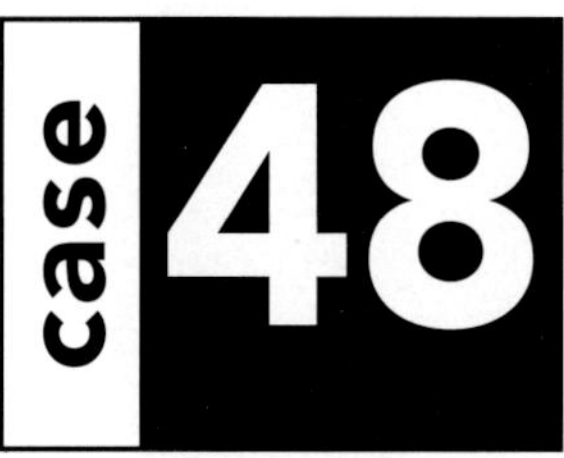

HISTORY

Mark Bright, a 70-year-old retired postman, was referred by his family doctor to Casualty for dehydration and a cough productive of purulent green sputum. He gave a history of cough productive of sputum for 5 days before his presentation.

For the past 6 weeks he had experienced nausea and regular vomiting which was particularly worse in the morning and after meals. There was no blood or bile in the vomitus. He had a history of recurrent, intermittent, upper abdominal pain that was worse before meals and radiated through to the back. The pain was relieved by antacids. He had noticed that his upper abdomen had become slightly distended. He had no appetite and he had lost nearly 5 kg in weight. He had also become constipated over the 4 weeks before presentation but was still passing flatus.

There was a history of lone atrial fibrillation controlled on digoxin. There was no family history of note. Other than digoxin, he took aspirin for occasional headache.

He smoked 15 cigarettes a day and denied drinking alcohol to excess.

Consider:

- **What are the causes of nausea and vomiting?**
- **Which organ system is the most likely cause of symptoms in this patient?**
- **How might the lone atrial fibrillation be associated with nausea and vomiting?**
- **What is the significance of the colour of the vomit?**

EXAMINATION

The patient was comfortable at rest. His tongue was dry and his eyes appeared sunken into the orbits. There was no jaundice, clubbing or lymphadenopathy.

His pulse was 100 beats/min irregularly irregular and his blood pressure was 120/70 mmHg supine with a pressure of 90/60 mmHg standing. His jugular venous pressure was not visible. His heart sounds revealed variable intensity of the first heart sound and there was an ejection systolic murmur over the aortic area that did not radiate.

Respiratory system examination revealed reduced expansion and reduced percussion note at the right. Auscultation of the lungs revealed crackles at the right base but a clear left lung.

Abdominal examination revealed a fullness in the epigastric region and palpation confirmed a mass in the epigastrium that was dull to percussion. On auscultation there was a succusion splash. Rectal examination was normal.

Examination of the central and peripheral nervous system was normal, in particular, there was absence of nystagmus and the eighth cranial nerve was normal.

Consider:

- **What is the relevance of the succussion splash?**
- **What is the likely cause of the lung disease?**

case 49

HISTORY

Milton P McCormick, a 25-year-old DIY enthusiast, had always been in good health. For the past 3 years, however, he had had a chronic low back pain which had started after an accident lifting weights in the gymnasium. The pain was episodic, had never radiated and was not accompanied by any lower limb numbness or paraesthesiae.

For some time he had planned to lay cork tiles in his kitchen. As his wife was going to be away for the weekend, he decided to carry out the whole work in her absence. By Sunday evening the job was completed. The work had involved spending much of the day kneeling, so that he could lay the tiles in place and cut them to size. His back pain had become rather worse and he took three aspirins before going to bed.

On getting out of bed the next morning, he realised that his right foot was moving awkwardly. It seemed to flop when he walked and on several occasions he had nearly tripped. He noticed no abnormal sensations in the leg and his left leg and foot seemed to be normal. His back pain had settled to its usual level. He took no immediate action but the problem persisted and he consulted his general practitioner 2 days later who advised a neurological opinion. He had no other neurological complaints at that time and his sphincter function was normal. Further enquiry by the general practitioner indicated that all was not well with the marriage, to the point where both partners had been considering a separation. Some of the patient's additional complaints suggested the probability of an anxiety state with depressive features. His sleep pattern had altered and he complained of feeling anxious and irritable during the day. He was finding it more difficult to concentrate at work and had become less enthusiastic about his DIY. He was a nonsmoker, seldom drank alcohol and took no medication apart from occasional analgesics.

Consider:

- **Could this be a stress-related problem?**
- **Does the distribution of the problem suggest organic neurological disease?**

EXAMINATION

His general systems examination was normal and the neurological abnormalities were confined to the right leg. His back movements appeared a little stiff and painful but straight leg raising was full. Proximal power in the right leg was normal. He had weakness of dorsiflexion of the foot (4/5) and of eversion (4/5). Extensor hallucis longus appeared rather more weak (3/5). Plantar flexion and inversion were intact. The reflexes were unremarkable and the plantars flexor bilaterally. There was possible blunting of cutaneous sensation over the dorsum of the right foot but proximal sensation, including the peri-anal region, was normal. When he walked, the right foot tended to drop and he had to lift the leg unnaturally at the hip to avoid tripping.

Consider:

- **Does the distribution of weakness suggest a particular nerve root or peripheral nerve disorder?**
- **What investigation would be of most value?**

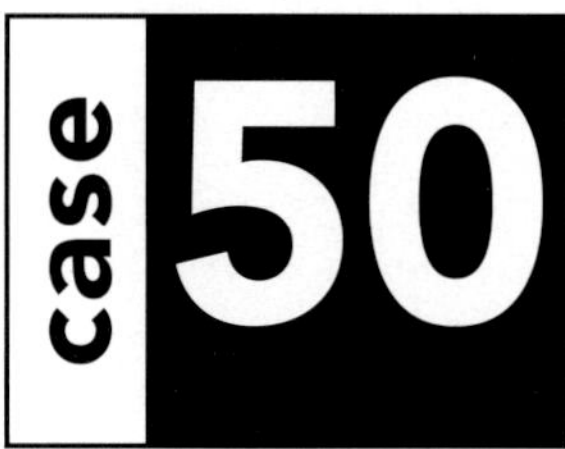

HISTORY

Anna Kelly, a 79-year-old woman, had dizzy spells and falls. She had had a series of blackouts that occurred without apparent warning. On at least one occasion she had fallen and injured herself. Her daughter said she went very pale as she lost consciousness and turned pink when she recovered. She had been taking atenolol for many years for high blood pressure.

Consider:
- **What are the likely causes of blackouts in this age group?**
- **Is there anything to point to a cardiac rather than a neurological cause in this history?**
- **What specific features should be looked for on examination?**

EXAMINATION

The patient looked alert and well for her age. Her pulse was 40 beats/min and regular. Her jugular venous pressure was normal. There was no clinical cardiac hypertrophy but there was a soft systolic murmur. Her blood pressure was 170/90 mmHg lying and standing. On gentle palpation the carotid pulse felt normal but the act of palpating it caused a further marked slowing of the pulse.

Consider:
- **What is the likely diagnosis?**
- **What are the possible causes of this condition?**
- **What investigations should be done?**

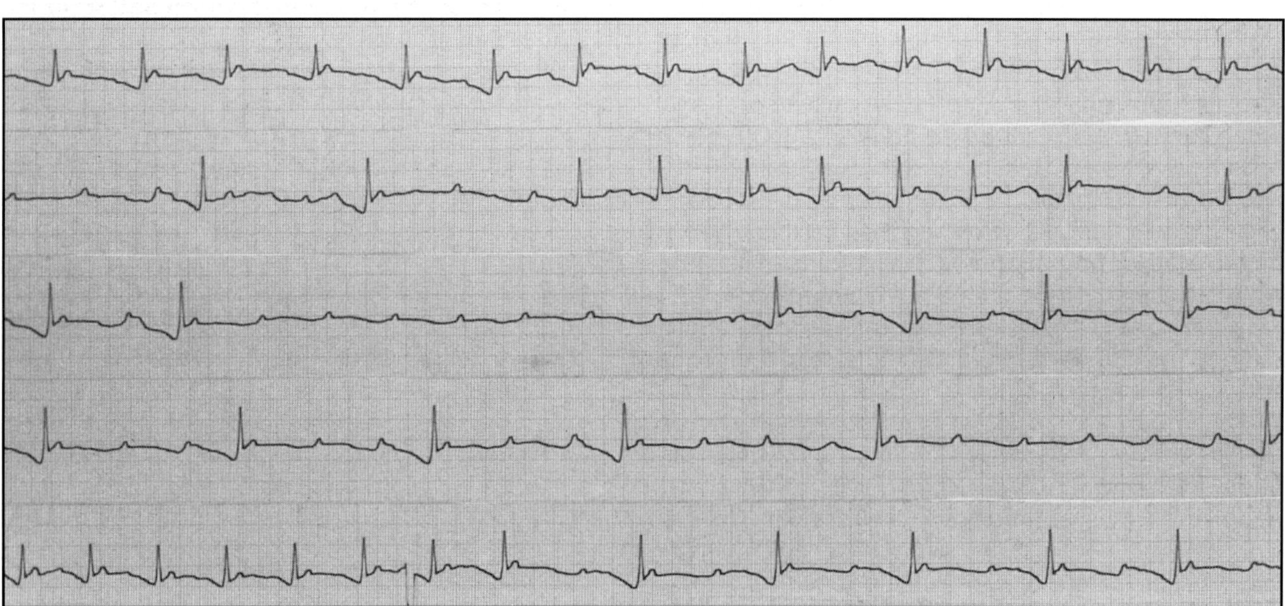

The patient's recordings from a 24-h ambulatory electrocardiogram.

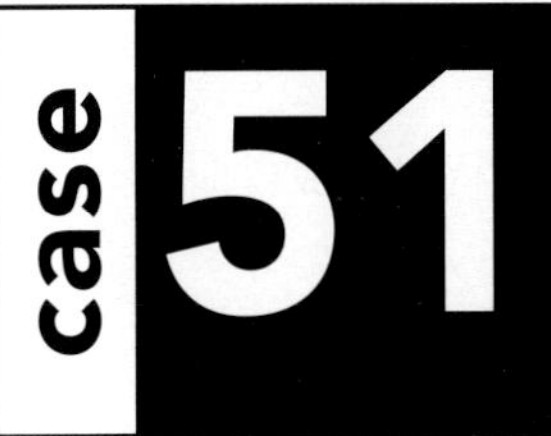

HISTORY

Lucile Lillywhite, a 24-year-old woman, had been well prior to her recent illness. She was unmarried but had a steady partner and was using a medium-strength (35 μg ethinyl oestradiol) mixed oral contraceptive. She worked as a secretary and spent much of her working day on a computer. Four days before seeking medical advice she had developed a pain in and above the left eye. The pain was quite substantial, with sharp components and was particularly evident when she looked to the left. Within 24 h, she had noticed a fogginess of her vision which she was certain was confined to the left eye. On the day of her consultation she had woken with very little vision in the eye apart from a slight awareness of movement and shapes in the periphery of her vision. She denied any other current symptoms and indicated that her general health was good. There was no family history of any visual complaint. She recalled that about a year before she had had some ill-defined parasthesiae in the peripheries of all four limbs which had lasted for approximately a month and then remitted. During that time she noticed that with neck flexion, a brief shock-like sensation had radiated down her spine into both lower limbs.

Consider:
- **What is the explanation for this patient's visual impairment?**
- **What is the significance of the symptoms a year before?**

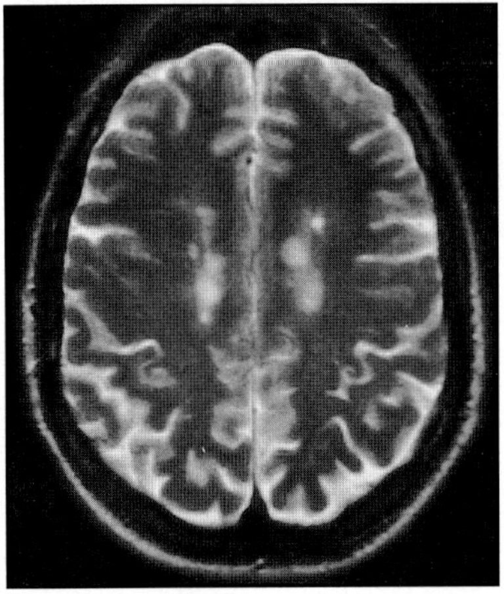

The patient's T2 weighted MRI scan.

EXAMINATION

On examination she appeared well but was anxious. The general systems examination was normal. Her visual acuities were 6/6 right and hand movements on the left. There was a left relative afferent pupillary defect. The left optic disc was slightly swollen with occasional peripapillary haemorrhages. The right optic disc appeared normal, with intact retinal venous pulsation. The visual field of the right eye was normal; that of the left was difficult to assess but there was a severe global reduction of vision perhaps maximal centrally. The rest of the cranial nerve examination was normal.

The limb reflexes were generally brisk with 2–3 beats of ankle clonus bilaterally. The plantars were flexor. The abdominal reflexes were absent. Limb power and tone appeared normal. Finger–nose and heel–knee–shin tests were well accomplished and her gait was unremarkable. Sensory testing was carried out for pain, light touch, joint position and vibration sense and was normal.

Within about a week the pain had resolved and by then she was confident of an improvement in her vision. She was beginning to recognise shapes in the central part of her vision although she had difficulty recognising their colour. By that time, her visual acuity had improved to 6/60 in the left eye.

Consider:
- **Has the examination confirmed the site of the problem causing visual impairment?**
- **Are there any other findings from the neurological examination that are significant?**
- **What is the working diagnosis?**
- **What would be the most valuable diagnostic procedure in this patient?**
- **What should you look for in the cerebrospinal fluid, if you decide to test it?**

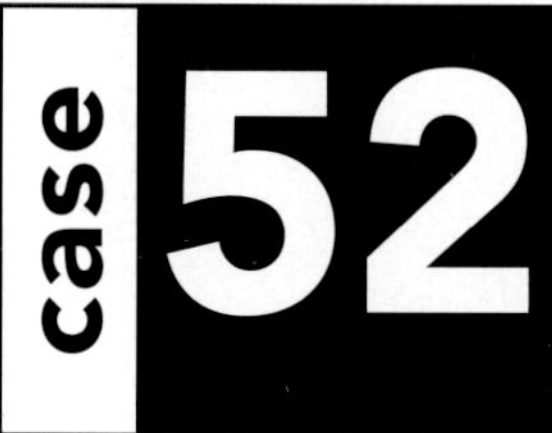

HISTORY

Reginald Walker-Taylor, a 56-year-old pilot, presented to the gastroenterlogy clinic with symptoms of blood in his stools and a change in his bowel habit. His bowels had been regular until 8 weeks previously after a flight to Bangkok. After the flight, he had noticed increased frequency and looser motions.

He became worried when he noticed the passage of blood and mucus mixed with the loose stool. The worry resulted in even more stool frequency with his bowel opening eight or nine times daily.

Three years previously he had experienced a single rectal bleed and his family doctor had diagnosed 'piles' which were treated with glycerine suppositories. He had taken codeine phosphate for the diarrhoea but without much success.

Nine months before presentation, he had been admitted to hospital for fevers and was successfully treated with antibiotics for *Streptococcus bovis* septicaemia. His health was otherwise normal. There was no family history of note.

The patient did not drink alcohol nor smoked. He took multivitamin tablets on a daily basis.

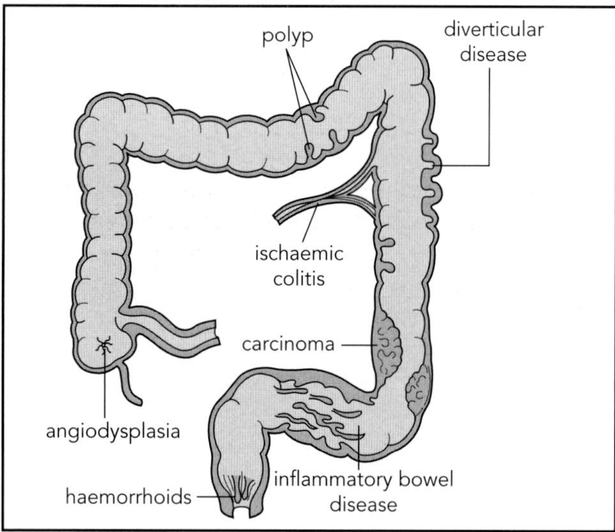

Colonic causes of blood in stool.

Consider:
- **Which of the above is the most likely cause of his bleeding, and why?**

EXAMINATION

The patient looked well and was well nourished. There was no jaundice, pallor or lymphadenopathy. His temperature was 37°C.

His pulse was 90 beats/min regular and of normal character. His blood pressure was 130/85 mmHg and his jugular venous pressure was not elevated. The first and second heart sounds were normal and there were no murmurs or other added sounds. His breath sounds were vesicular.

On abdominal palpation there was an irregular, hard liver edge palpable 5 cm below the right costal margin. No other masses were palpable within the abdomen. His bowel sounds were normal. Rectal examination was normal as was a proctoscopy and rigid sigmoidoscopy.

Neurological examination was normal.

Consider:
- **What is the relevance of the enlarged liver?**
- **What investigations would provide a diagnosis?**

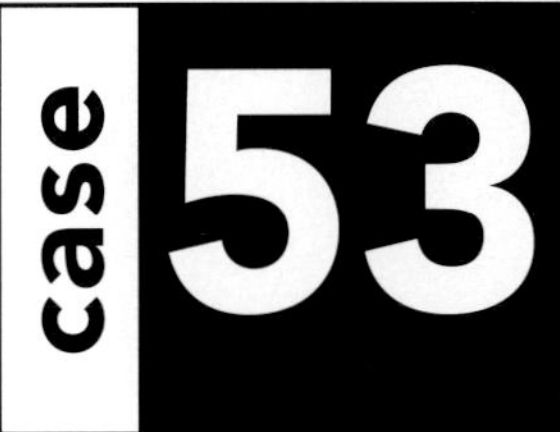

HISTORY

Yasmin Dubois, a 74-year-old woman, had been admitted to hospital as an emergency several days previously, since then she had started to feel a little better. She had been assessed by the admitting team as being in cardiac failure; her diuretic treatment had been increased and an angiotensin-converting enzyme inhibitor added. She confirmed that she had been admitted to hospital several times in the past 2 years with the same problems. On further questioning, it was established that she had been short of breath for approximately 5 years but she was not unduly troubled by this until she developed a sudden worsening of the breathlessness accompanied by swelling of the ankles approximately 2 years previously. Although she improved every time she was admitted, she remained persistently short of breath in between and had not been able to shop independently or do much housework for approximately 18 months. There was little variation in her symptoms from day to day. She had a cough productive of occasional sputum and she had some wheeze, especially when she was breathless. She had had no chest pain. She slept well but had been unable to sleep lying flat for years.

She had no previous health problems. She had smoked 60 cigarettes a day and had been unable to give up despite the exhortations of her doctors. She was employed for many years as an office cleaner. Although she was pleased that the diuretics helped the ankle swelling, she was uncertain whether they helped with her breathing.

Consider:
- **What is the alternative diagnosis to heart failure?**
- **What should be looked for on examination?**

EXAMINATION

The patient appeared breathless even at rest but was able to talk in sentences. She appeared centrally cyanosed but her oxygen mask was around her neck instead of fixed securely over her face. There was no clubbing or lymphadenopathy but there was marked ankle and sacral oedema. In the cardiovascular system examination, her pulse rate was 105 beats/min,,she was in sinus rhythm and her blood pressure was 115/85 mmHg. Her jugular venous pulse appeared to be moving her earlobes with a prominent 'V' wave. The apex beat could not be located but there was a left parasternal heave. There was a short systolic murmur and a third sound heard over the precordium.

In the respiratory system examination, the trachea was central, expansion equal but reduced and the percussion note normal. On auscultation the breath sounds were rather poor in all areas and there was some end-expiratory wheeze and a few rather coarse basal crackles occurring early in inspiration. In the abdomen, her liver was enlarged 5 cm below the costal margin and was pulsatile.

During the examination, the patient complained of headache and by the end she had become drowsy and incoherent.

Consider:
- **What is the significance of the cardiovascular system findings?**
- **How has the examination contributed to an understanding of this patient's problem?**
- **What has happened to her during the examination?**

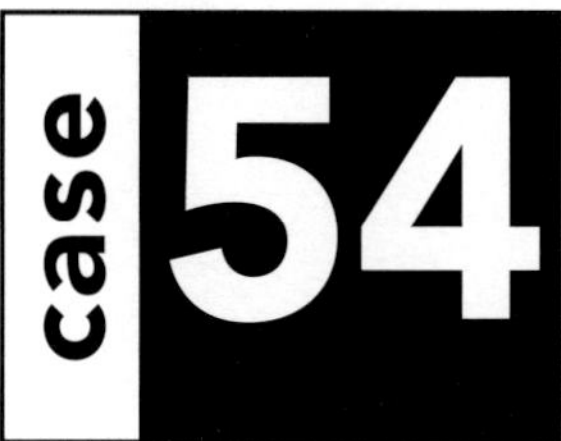

HISTORY

Angela John, a 35-year-old legal secretary, consulted her family doctor 2 weeks ago complaining of a 6-week history of fatigue, fever and diarrhoea. She had also noticed some shortness of breath while shopping which had never previously troubled her.

The doctor suggested a course of penicillin for her symptoms and treated her for a chest infection.

However, she returned a week later no better, complaining of painful shins and an nonproductive cough. Her family doctor decided to refer her to the local hospital for a specialist opinion.

In the course of repeating her history, she mentioned that she had asthma as a child and she kept a budgie that was healthy. There was no known family history other than her father and both her sisters having mild psoriasis. Other than the penicillin prescribed by her family doctor she was taking the oral contraceptive pill.

Consider:

- **What are the causes of breathlessness?**
- **Is the budgie of relevance?**
- **Does the diarrhoea influence the differential diagnosis?**

EXAMINATION

The patient gave the appearance of looking unwell. She had a temperature of 37.5°C. There was no lymphadenopathy or clubbing.

Her pulse was 80 beats/min regular and of normal character. Her blood pressure was 120/80 mmHg and her jugular venous pressure was not visible. The first and second heart sounds were normal without any additional heart sounds and there was no peripheral oedema.

Examination of the respiratory system revealed a respiratory rate of 18 breaths/min. The expansion was reduced bilaterally and symmetrically. Percussion note was normal. The breath sounds were vesicular but with fine inspiratory crackles at the lung bases.

Abdominal and rectal examination, as well as the central nervous system examination, were normal.

Examination of the lower limbs revealed painful erythematous nodules over the shins.

Consider:

- **Is the penicillin a possible cause of the skin lesion?**
- **What is the most likely cause of the lung disorder?**
- **What is the skin disorder?**

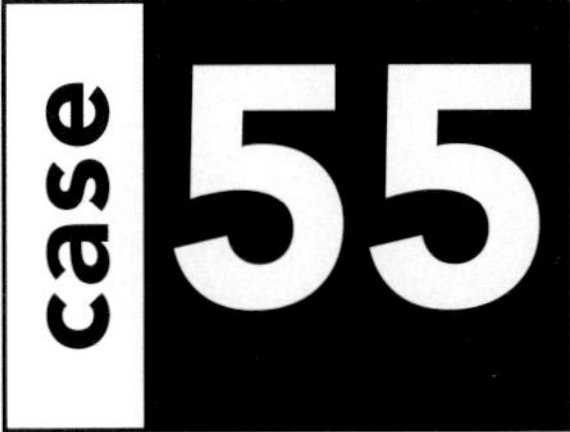

case 55

HISTORY

Daniel Darling, a 78-year-old retired diplomat, had travelled extensively in the Middle East before his retirement at the age of 60 years. He had not been abroad in recent years, being restricted by osteoarthritis of the hips. He had had bilateral hip joint replacements that had only been moderately successful. He lived with his wife who was in good health. He was a nonsmoker but drank regularly, probably averaging 30–35 units per week.

One week before, he had developed a pain in the region of the left mastoid process associated with irritation in the left ear. The pain had intensified and he had required regular analgesics. Two days before the consultation, he had realised that fluids were tending to dribble from the left angle of his mouth. His wife had accused him of drinking as his speech appeared slurred. On looking in the mirror, he realised he could not completely close his left eye. At about the same time he noticed that noises were exaggerated in the left ear. He felt that his sense of taste had altered and that it was defective on the left side of the tongue. His balance had perhaps slightly deteriorated but he denied vertigo. He had no other neurological complaints. Generally he felt less well than normal, although he could not specify any particular complaint. He was on no medication apart from low dose aspirin which his general practitioner had advised after a possible minor heart attack 3 years previously.

Consider:
- **What type of facial palsy is suggested by the history?**
- **What is the significance of the altered taste and the hyperacusis?**

EXAMINATION

On examination he appeared reasonably well, although clearly dispirited by his recent symptoms. A general systems examination was unremarkable. He had a blood pressure of 158/88 mmHg and he was in sinus rhythm. His range of hip movements was restricted bilaterally and his gait was a little clumsy.

His fundi were normal and eye movements intact. Facial sensation was normal and his jaw muscles appeared of normal power. He failed to blink with his left eye and its palpebral fissure was widened compared with the right. The sclera of the left eye was slightly injected. There was loss of furrowing of the left forehead and a failure of elevation of the eyebrow. There was striking weakness of the lower face on the left; the right was normal. Crude testing of taste suggested it was impaired over the left side of the tongue anteriorly. He was hypersensitive to noise in the left ear. Hearing in the right ear was normal. There was a focal area of redness with scab formation in the left external auditory meatus and a similar area in the region of the left hard palate. The rest of the neurological examination was normal.

Consider:
- **Has the examination confirmed the nature of the facial palsy?**
- **What is the significance of the rash in the ear and throat?**
- **What might be found if the patient's spinal fluid was examined?**
- **What precautions might be needed to avoid any complication of this facial weakness and what outcome would be expected?**

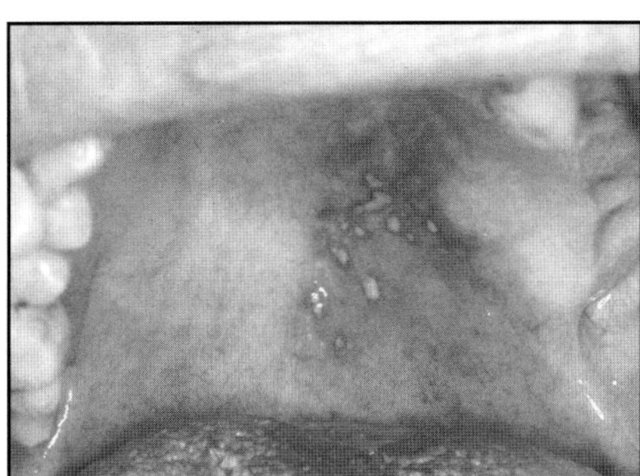

The patient's palate.

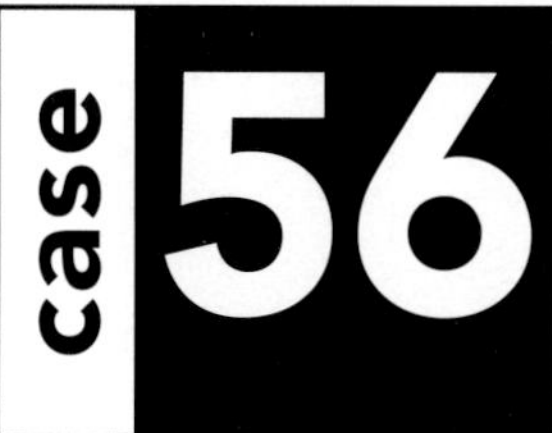

HISTORY

Nicola Simpson, a 34-year-old housewife with two daughters, complained of lethargy and tiredness 2 months after her second pregnancy. The pregnancy had been uncomplicated but the third stage of labout was problematic and she required a 2 unit blood transfusion because of blood loss. Her doctor wondered if she was suffering from postnatal depression and managed her with counselling. However there was no improvement in her symptoms.

Four months into the postpartum period, the patient still had not begun her periods and was becoming concerned. She also noted that she would lose her hair every morning on combing. She did not complain of a headache. She felt 'cold'.

On questioning she also described a change in her bowel habit tending towards constipation. She also commented on her failure to produce breast milk as well as urinary frequency.

Before her second pregnancy she had enjoyed good health. This pregnancy had been uncomplicated until labour which was prolonged and associated with excessive bleeding and during which she required transfusion of three units of blood.

There was no family history and she was not taking any medication at the time of presentation. She denied drinking alcohol in excess and did not smoke.

Consider:
- **What is the likely cause of her symptoms?**
- **Why has she noticed increased urinary frequency?**
- **What probably caused the disease?**
- **Why did she fail to lactate?**

EXAMINATION

On general examination the patient appeared pale and unwell. There was sparse axillary hair and pubic hair. There was no jaundice, clubbing or lymphadenopathy. There were wrinkles around her mouth.

On examination of the cardiovascular system her pulse was 90 beats/min regular but low volume. The blood pressure was 100/70 mmHg supine with a postural drop of 30 mmHg. Her jugular venous pressure was not elevated. The first and second heart sounds were normal. There was no peripheral oedema. The breath sounds were vesicular and examination of the abdomen was normal.

Examination of the neurological system revealed weakness in the proximal muscles and slow relaxing reflexes. Examination of the cranial nerves was normal and there were no visual field defects or papilloedema.

Consider:
- **What is the relevance of the hair loss?**
- **Why does she have postural hypeotension?**
- **Why did she look pale?**

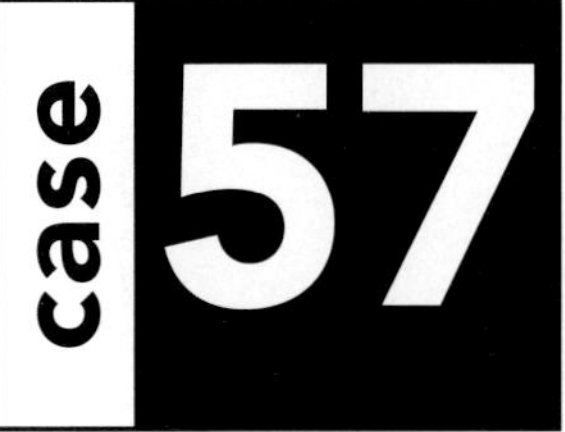

HISTORY

Christy de Winter, a 35-year-old woman, had had a stressful time over the previous 2 years. For some time she had complained of diffuse pains in her body but particularly in her shoulders and hands. She had been working on a computer and her general practitioner had diagnosed repetitive strain injury, even though the symptoms were very symmetrical. Her company's doctor had advised her to switch occupations and she had been under considerable pressure from her company to do so, particularly as her work output had suffered. A year before, she had become pregnant; although she had a long-term partner, she had not contemplated having children but decided to proceed with the pregnancy. She left her work. During the pregnancy her pains had improved substantially but her problems worsened soon after delivery. She began to wake with considerable stiffness in her hands that could take up to 2 h to settle. She noticed that her pains were now concentrated in the knuckles in both hands which at times, to her, appeared slightly swollen and tender. At times she noticed pains in the left wrist and right elbow. She felt generally unwell and had increased her cigarette consumption from 10 to 20 a day. She denied other specific symptoms, although she admitted her problems had caused her to become increasingly irritable and this had resulted in some strain in the relationship with her partner. She had taken aspirin periodically and had found it to be of some benefit in pain control. She was on no other medication and seldom drank alcohol. The family history was unremarkable, as was the systems review.

Consider:

- **Has this patient an organic disease or could the whole problem be stress-related?**
- **What type of process, if this is organic, underlies her symptoms?**
- **What is the most likely diagnosis?**

EXAMINATION

The general examination was unremarkable, although the patient appeared anxious and tired. Abnormalities were confined to the upper limbs. There appeared to be a slight reduction of extension of the right elbow. Attempts to move the joint further caused pain. Similarly, extension of the left wrist appeared slightly limited with some swelling in the region of the ulnar styloid. Mild swelling of the metacarpophalangeal and proximal interphalangeal joints was apparent and was symmetrical. The joints were slightly tender to palpation. The patient had difficulty in making a fist and complained of reduced grip strength, although much of the problem appeared to be caused by pain.

Consider:

- **Has the examination settled the issue of organic disease?**
- **What investigations might support the diagnosis?**
- **How can the problem be managed?**

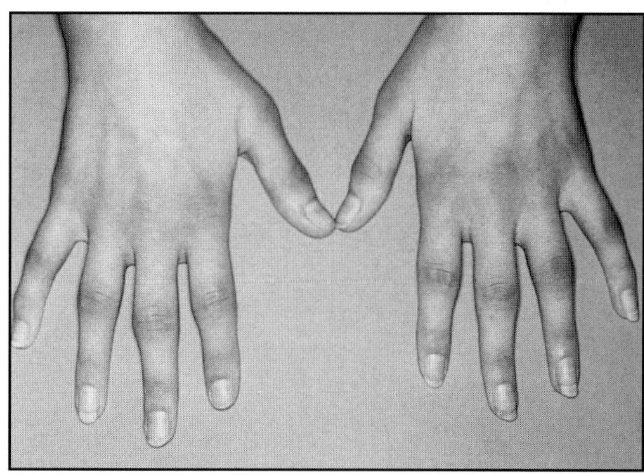

The patient's hands.

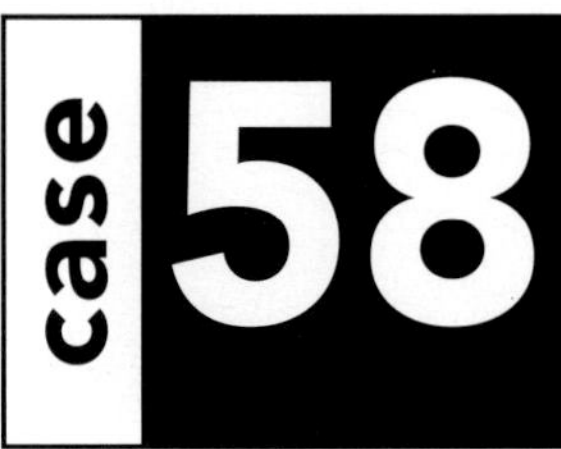

HISTORY

Frederick Thompson, a 65-year-old man, presented with shortness of breath. The symptom was progressive over a 2-month period and he found difficulty shopping and walking up an incline, although there was little breathlessness while he was at home.

Six months previously he had been admitted to hospital with a single episode of unstable angina that had not progressed to a myocardial infarct. He had smoked 20 cigarettes daily for 30 years but had stopped smoking at the time of admission.

After the ischaemic event he had been advised to increase the amount of fatty fish in his diet and he had been prescribed a ß blocker and a daily dose of soluble aspirin (150 mg).

Condider:

- **What is the likely origin of the symptom and why?**
- **What is the most likely diagnosis and why?**
- **What examinations should be carried out?**

EXAMINATION

The patient was not short of breath at rest. His pulse was 56 beats/min, regular and of normal character. His blood pressure was 120/70 mmHg and he had conjunctival pallor. Jugular venous pressure was not visualised.

On examination of his chest the apex beat was not displaced and, on auscultation, the first and second heart sounds were normal. However, there was a soft aortic ejection murmur in the second right intercostal space that did not radiate to the carotids.

On examination of the lungs there was good respiratory movement. There was normal percussion and, on auscultation, there were a few rhonchi that cleared with coughing. The abdominal and neurological examinations were normal

Consider:

- **Has the examination helped clarify the initial differential diagnosis?**
- **Are there any predisposing factors from the history?**
- **Are there any complications?**

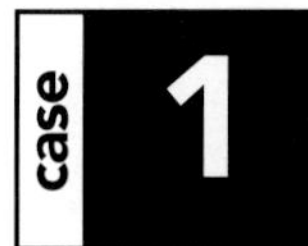

DIFFERENTIAL DIAGNOSIS

1. Cavernous aneurysm
2. Chordoma
3. Meningioma

DISCUSSION

The lesion is most likely to be in the region of the cavernous sinus on the basis of the history. The oculomotor nerve has been affected from the beginning. Although there is some abduction of the left eye, it is incomplete, indicating a partial abducens palsy. With the eye abducted as far as possible, there is no rotatory twitch on attempted down gaze, indicating involvement of the trochlear nerve. In other words, all the oculomotor nerves of the left eye are affected. In addition, there is a definite involvement of the first division of the trigeminal nerve and possible involvement of the second division. The other cranial nerves are spared.

The lesion is unlikely to be in the orbit because of the only equivocal proptosis and the probable involvement of the second division of the trigeminal nerve. For this latter reason, the lesion is also unlikely to be in the superior orbital fissure. The problem is likely to be in the mid to anterior aspect of the cavernous sinus.

From what appears to be a compressive lesion in the cavernous sinus, and from what is virtually a complete third nerve palsy, you would have expected the left pupil to be dilated rather than comparable in size to the right. The similarity in size suggests that the sympathetic fibres to the left pupil are also damaged.

The most likely diagnosis is a giant cavernous aneurysm. These fusiform aneurysms are degenerative and linked to hypertension. They tend to expand gradually and are typically painful. They also occur on the basilar artery. They seldom rupture, exerting their effect by local pressure.

Management of these cases is extremely difficult and usually has to be conservative. The aneurysm cannot be approached directly by surgery. Ligation of the feeding carotid artery in the neck tends to have a very limited effect on the growth of the aneurysm and is not without hazard.

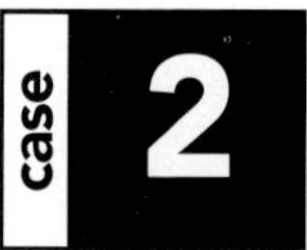

DIFFERENTIAL DIAGNOSIS

1. Diffuse oesophageal spasm
2. Cardiac pain, either angina or myocardial infarction
3. Aortic dissection

DISCUSSION

The history is of recurrent retrosternal chest pain in an overweight smoker. Retrosternal chest pain usually has three causes: cardiac, oesophageal or, more rarely, aortic dissection.

A cardiac cause is unlikely because the pains have occurred at rest, without a previous history of exertional chest pain. Furthermore, the patient's electrocardiogram is normal during an episode of pain.

An aortic dissection should always be considered with a history of retrosternal chest pain, particularly if it radiates to the back. However, aortic dissection is unlikely because of the previous similar episodes of pain that have resolved spontaneously without ill effect. The patient does not have any clinical signs suggestive of aortic dissection (unequal pulses, differing blood pressure in either arm, murmur of aortic incompetence, widened mediastinum on chest radiograph). Aortic dissection can be present without these clinical signs and, if seriously suspected, transoesophageal echocardiography or a computerised tomography scan should be considered.

The history is suggestive of an oesophageal cause. Diffuse oesophageal spasm can mimic the pain of cardiac ischaemia but tends to occur at rest or after a large meal. It can be associated with dysphagia. The pain may be relieved with sublingual nitrates which may add to the difficulty in discriminating the pain from a cardiac source. The pain can vary from a mild discomfort that lasts a few seconds to a severe and prolonged episode. The pain is often confused with cardiac pain and can be severe enough to mimic a myocardial infarct. Gastro-oesophageal acid reflux is a common cause of diffuse oesophageal spasm.

This patient has diffuse oesophageal spasm caused by gastro-oesophageal reflux. He described preceding indigestion pains that may have been precipitated by the recent tricyclic antidepressant. Tricyclic antidepressants (via their anticholinergic effects) lower the pressure in the lower oesophageal sphincter which can exacerbate acid reflux. The patient is also overweight and a smoker which are predisposing factors for both acid reflux and myocardial ischaemia.

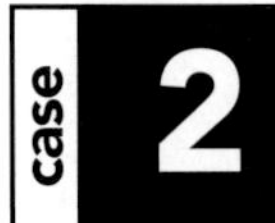

Other predisposing factors for acid reflux include caffeine or chocolate ingestion and pregnancy.

Diffuse oesophageal spasm, if suspected, is most usefully investigated by barium swallow or oesophageal manometry. If acid reflux is suspected, then endoscopy may show oesophagitis. Occasionally, the symptoms of acid reflux may be difficult to elucidate; performing a 24-h oesophageal pH study may help the diagnosis.

The treatment of diffuse oesophageal spasm remains difficult. If acid reflux is a factor, then treating this with a H_2 antagonist or a proton-pump inhibitor can help symptoms. Treatment of the oesophageal spasm with calcium-channel blockers or nitrates is used with variable benefit. Reassuring the patient that the pains are not cardiac often helps. Severe intractable problems with oesophageal spasm can be treated surgically with a myotomy but this is reserved in most centres as a last measure.

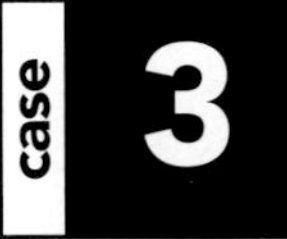

DIFFERENTIAL DIAGNOSIS

1. Multiple sclerosis
2. Cervical spondylosis with myelopathy
3. Spinal cord angioma

DISCUSSION

This patient has a progressive spastic paraparesis on the basis of the history. There were no previous neurological events. The symptoms appear to be exacerbated by exercise. Although the patient's symptoms and signs are largely motor, she has evidence of an unstable bladder and has sensory abnormalities on physical examination.

Vitamin B_{12} deficiency (a very unlikely diagnosis) has been excluded. The negative computerised tomography scan has essentially excluded a parasagittal meningioma which was not particularly likely on the basis of her history. She has no history nor physical findings to suggest cervical myelopathy caused by disc disease. Spinal meningiomas (which are usually thoracic) predominate in women and it is conceivable that this is the underlying pathology. The gradually evolving symmetrical picture and the exercise-induced symptoms, however, favour multiple sclerosis as the diagnosis.

Cerebrospinal fluid examination would not be the first choice of investigation here. If there was only an elevated protein concentration, the other tests being normal, then a meningioma would remain a possible diagnosis. If the cerebrospinal fluid showed oligoclonal bands, then the diagnosis of multiple sclerosis would be strongly supported.

It would probably be best to start with magnetic resonance imaging of the cervical and thoracic cord. A meningioma would then be readily identified, as would virtually all cases of spinal angioma. The cord may show abnormal signal areas or be simply atrophic if the diagnosis was multiple sclerosis. If the spinal magnetic resonance imaging is unhelpful, brain magnetic resonance imaging is likely to show the signal changes associated with multiple sclerosis.

It would be worth trying an antispastic agent, such as baclofen, although the drug is unlikely to aid the major problem of exercise-induced weakness. She probably has sphincter–detrusor dyssynergia and may well benefit from the use of oxybutynin.

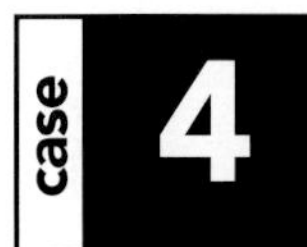

DIFFERENTIAL DIAGNOSIS

1. Acute pericarditis
2. Pleurisy
3. Myocardial ischaemia

DISCUSSION

An electrocardiogram showed saddle-shaped ST elevation in all leads. The haemoglobin was 10.9 and plasma viscosity was elevated. A chest radiograph was normal.

Echocardiography showed good left ventricular function with a small pericardial effusion. A diagnosis of acute pericarditis was made and she was treated symptomatically with ibuprofen pending further investigation.

Twenty-four hours later she became breathless and shocked with a raised jugular venous pressure. Echocardiography showed an enlarging effusion with tamponade that required pericardial aspiration. A dilute Mantoux test was strongly positive and mycobacterium tuberculosis was eventually grown from the pericardial aspirate.

Although the initial history very strongly suggests pericarditis, the differential diagnosis would include pleurisy, for example, from pulmonary embolism or myocardial ischaemia (the patient smoked and was on the pill).

The finding of a pericardial rub strongly suggests pericarditis but this sign is often intermittent and commonly disappears with the development of a pericardial effusion.

Causes of pericarditis include viral and bacterial infection, autoimmune disease (e.g. systemic lupus erythematosus) and uraemia.

Primary tuberculous pericarditis is not uncommon where tuberculosis is endemic and may have been acquired during the patient's visit to India. The normal chest radiograph does not exclude the diagnosis. The prognosis is good with appropriate antibiotic treatment but a proportion of patients go on to develop constrictive pericarditis.

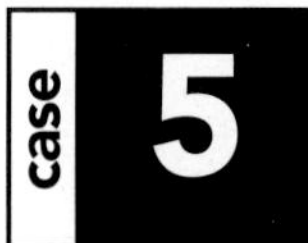

DIFFERENTIAL DIAGNOSIS

1. Parkinson's disease
2. Multisystem atrophy
3. Progressive supranuclear palsy

DISCUSSION

The physical examination revealed evidence of a symmetrical syndrome of rigidity combined with bradykinesia in the absence of tremor. It is sensible to describe this as an akinetic rigid syndrome rather than immediately assume that the condition is one of idiopathic Parkinson's disease. Of every 100 patients with a reasonably confident diagnosis of Parkinson's disease, only approximately 75 are found to have the condition at postmortem examination.

Features that suggest this is unlikely to be idiopathic Parkinson's disease include the presence of sphincter disturbance at an early stage in the illness and both the history and examination findings of possible postural hypotension. All these features suggest autonomic involvement and raise the question of multisystem atrophy.

Conventional imaging techniques will not be helpful in the investigation. Electromyography of the urinary sphincter shows denervation in the vast majority of patients with multisystem atrophy. Formal assessment of autonomic function may well give equivocal results at this stage but later, profound postural hypotension is likely, together with evidence of hypersensitivity to infusions of noradrenaline or tyramine.

Some patients with multisystem atrophy respond to dopa, although the majority do not. A negative response to therapy will, however, point the diagnosis away from idiopathic Parkinson's disease and towards multisystem atrophy.

The patient must be advised to get out of bed slowly in the morning, sitting on the edge for several minutes before standing. He should micturate in the sitting position, particularly at night. If he develops dizziness, he should sit down immediately. Although various drugs have been tried for the postural hypotension of multisystem atrophy, their effect is very limited.

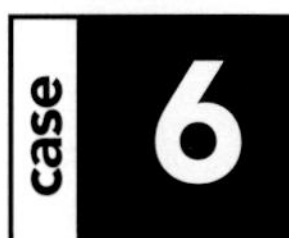

DIFFERENTIAL DIAGNOSIS

1. First febrile convulsion with upper respiratory infection
2. First epileptic fit with a fever
3. Meningitis and encephalitis appear to be unlikely

DISCUSSION

Febrile convulsions are common in preschool age children (approximately 3–4% of children under 5 years of age). They are also very distressing for parents to witness, 'I thought my child was dying' is a common quote given by parents in the history. Happily the prognosis is very good; most children (>60%) will not have another convulsion. The risk gets much less by the age of 3 years.

Approximately 1% of what present as 'febrile convulsions' are in fact a child's first fit precipitated by fever. These children go on to have more fits, with and without fevers, and have true epilepsy. The prognosis in these patients is variable.

The absence of neck stiffness, a negative Kernig's sign and a normal level of consciousness make central nervous system infection very unlikely. In children under 2 years of age, and especially under 1 year of age, signs of meningeal irritation are not always present in meningitis. Hence, with children under 24 months, there needs to be a lower threshold for lumbar puncture to rule out central nervous system infection. In this two-and-a-half-year-old, it is therefore unlikely to be central nervous system infection.

The management includes admitting him for observation and providing information and reassurance to the parents about febrile convulsions. When his fever lessens and his parents have regained their confidence, they can all go home.

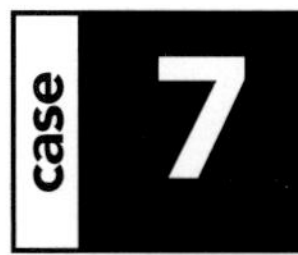

DIFFERENTIAL DIAGNOSIS

1. Chest infection: pneumonia and pleurisy
2. Pulmonary embolism
3. Chest wall pain

DISCUSSION

This case illustrates a common clinical dilemma: that of distinguishing an uncommon but serious condition, pulmonary embolism, from a common but usually benign condition, pulmonary infection. Sometimes the presentation is clear cut but often the picture is confused.

In this patient pulmonary embolism is suggested by the recent surgery, the sudden onset of pain and the possible haemoptysis. Predisposing factors include smoking and perhaps a minor effect from hormone replacement therapy. Against the diagnosis is the lack of significant breathlessness and of any symptoms of a deep vein thrombosis, although the latter is present in only a minority.

Infection is suggested by the general anaesthetic, the cold, cough and yellow sputum. Smoking would predispose to infection.

Chest wall pain needs to be borne in mind as muscle damage or even rib fracture can follow from prolonged coughing bouts, and the patient did suggest that there was a tender area.

The examination is of limited value. The lack of a localised tenderness makes chest wall pain unlikely. The slight tachycardia could be a response to fever, indicate some cardiac problem or merely be due to anxiety. Mild fever and a pleural rub are possible in both infection and infarction. The lack of evidence of right heart strain (raised jugular venous pressure and a right ventricular third sound) or of a deep vein thrombosis makes a large embolism unlikely.

The most likely cause of the patient's problem is infection but there is sufficient circumstantial evidence of pulmonary embolism that this diagnosis needs to be formally excluded.

The chest radiograph is often normal in pulmonary embolism whereas consolidation would be characteristic of pneumonia. Blood gases are likely to be disturbed in both and show hypoxia and a lowered partial pressure of carbon dioxide. A lung scan should show unmatched defects in pulmonary embolism but matched ones in pneumonia but the technique may not be diagnostic. In difficult cases, a pulmonary arteriogram may be required.

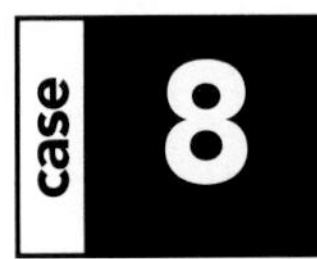

DIFFERENTIAL DIAGNOSIS

1. Terminal ileal disease: inflammatory bowel disease or, more rarely, tuberculosis or lymphoma
2. Irritable bowel syndrome
2. Caecal carcinoma
3. Appendicular abscess
4. Gynaecological causes including ovarian cyst or carcinoma or salpingitis

DISCUSSION

The history details right iliac fossa pain associated with general malaise, weight loss and minor change of bowel habit. When taking a history for abdominal pain it is important to document precisely its localisation, character, aggravating or relieving factors and other visceral symptoms. Eliciting these factors will aid in reaching a diagnosis.

The differential diagnosis of right iliac fossa pain lies between gynaecological and small or large bowel disorders. There is no menstrual disturbance and no relationship between the pain and menstruation. This makes gynaecological causes less likely (but does not rule them out). Common bowel causes of right iliac fossa pain in young patients normally involve irritable bowel syndrome or inflammatory bowel disease. Irritable bowel syndrome is unlikely as weight loss and pain waking the patient from sleep is not characteristic. A caecal carcinoma would be unusual but not unheard of in this age group. One would expect the patient to be more unwell with an appendicular abscess.

The important finding on clinical examination is the small tender lump on the patient's lower limb. This description is compatible with erythema nodosum which commonly occurs on the shins. There are a number of causes of erythema nodosum including idiopathic, inflammatory bowel disease, streptococcal infection, drug reactions (oral contraceptive pill, sulphonamides, barbiturates), sarcoidosis and tuberculosis.

The combination of right iliac fossa pain, malaise, weight loss, change of bowel habit and erythema nodosum in a young patient is highly suggestive of Crohn's disease. Young patients with inflammatory bowel disease may look surprisingly well even during episodes of significant disease activity. A change of bowel habit is not always seen in small bowel Crohn's disease.

Erythema nodosum is an extra-intestinal manifestation of inflammatory bowel disease. Clinical examination of a patient with inflammatory bowel disease should involve careful inspection of the mouth and perianal areas in addition to a more generalised examination. Other organs involved in inflammatory bowel disease include the eyes (uveitis, episcleritis, conjunctivitis), liver (fatty change, pericholangitis, sclerosing cholangitis, cirrhosis), joints (ankylosing spondylitis, monoarticular arthritis), skin (erythema nodosum, pyoderma gangrenosum) and kidney or renal stones.

Once Crohn's disease is suspected, initial investigations usually involve routine blood tests. During disease activity these will often show a rise in 'inflammatory markers' such as raised white blood cell and platelet count, raised erythrocyte sedimentation rate or C-reactive protein. Haematinics should be requested particularly to detect B_{12} deficiency (the terminal ileum being the site of its absorption). A well-performed barium meal and follow through will detect small bowel disease. Treatment involves immunosuppression usually in the form of corticosteroids and 5-aminosalicylic acid compounds.

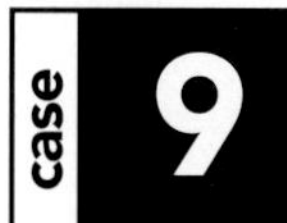

case 9

DIFFERENTIAL DIAGNOSIS

1. Myasthenia gravis

DISCUSSION

The history is strongly suggestive of myasthenia gravis. There is an association between that condition and other auto-immune disorders, including thyrotoxicosis. Typically, the patient's symptoms fluctuate, as is the case here, in which there is a strong suggestion of fatiguability of the singing voice. When myasthenic patients complain of diplopia, it is often difficult to pinpoint the affected muscle or muscles which may well vary during the course of the consultation. Often the fluctuant quality of the limb power performance is attributed to the patient being uncooperative.

A formal assessment of fatiguability should be carried out. The patient can be asked to look upwards for, say, a minute, to see whether any ptosis increases. They can be asked to count to 100 to assess speech and then asked to abduct the arms at the shoulders for a minute to assess fatiguability of the deltoids.

The tensilon test is recommended as a pharmacological test, although it is not without hazard. In patients already on anticholinesterases, an increase in weakness from the injection due to a cholinergic crisis can lead to respiratory arrest. Rarely, the injection can cause an asystolic cardiac arrest from enhancement of vagal tone. A test dose of 2 mg intravenously is given, followed by 8 mg, during which any ptosis or other obvious weakness is assessed.

Measurement of acetylcholine receptor antibodies is the most helpful blood test. The clinical picture suggests the patient has generalised myasthenia and you would expect to find the antibodies in at least 90% of such cases.

You should consider imaging the patient's thymus. Exclusion of a thymoma is particularly important because thymectomy would be needed. The more likely finding would be evidence of thymic hyperplasia. Although a simple chest radiograph can detect many thymomas, the investigation of choice is computerised tomography of the mediastinum.

case 10

DIFFERENTIAL DIAGNOSIS

1. Heart failure
2. Lung disease
3. Ischaemic heart disease

DISCUSSION

Breathlessness is a common presenting symptom and it is possible to approach it in a systematic way. Common causes of breathlessness in a man of this age include heart failure, lung disease and, less commonly, ischaemic heart disease presenting without angina, pulmonary embolism or anaemia. The gradual onset of symptoms and their duration point to a chronic rather than an acute cause. The patient is describing the symptom of orthopnoea: an inability to lie flat comfortably. This is a feature pointing to heart failure. The presence of peripheral but not central cyanosis would tilt the diagnosis towards a cardiac rather than a lung cause. The most common cause of pitting ankle oedema in elderly people is stasis rather than heart failure but in this patient the oedema is more extensive.

The electrocardiogram showed sinus rhythm with left bundle branch block and the chest radiograph showed an enlarged heart but no pulmonary oedema. Echocardiography showed a dilated, poorly contracting, left ventricle with no pericardial effusion and no valve abnormalities. The patient improved on treatment with a diuretic and an angiotensin-converting enzyme inhibitor.

Heart failure is a common condition affecting between 1% and 2% of the UK population. The most common causes are hypertension and ischaemic heart disease. In this patient, there may have been a background of high blood pressure and his measured blood pressure of 150/100 mmHg perhaps suggests this. However, low blood pressure is not a characteristic feature of chronic heart failure. Although the initial damage was almost certainly done to the left ventricle, there is also little evidence of pulmonary oedema. This is because the gradual development of left heart failure allows compensation by pulmonary vasoconstriction and the final picture is one of biventricular or 'congestive' heart failure. Nonsteroidal anti-inflammatory drugs such as indomethacin are commonly prescribed. They can exacerbate hypertension and cause salt and water retention.

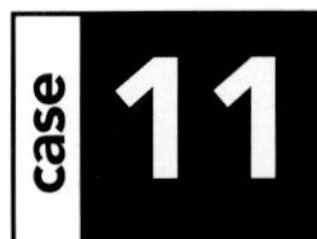

DISCUSSION

The clinical history suggests the presence of a bulbar palsy. The afferent part of the gag reflex (elicited by stimulating the tonsillar fossa with firm pressure from an orange stick) is supplied by the glossopharyngeal nerve. The efferent part of the reflex (palatal elevation) is supplied by the vagus. Where there is a unilateral palatal palsy, the palate deviates to the intact side. The sternomastoid muscle and the upper fibres of trapezius are supplied by the accessory nerve. The combined findings in this patient therefore (excluding those attributable to his AIDS-related dementia) point to a lesion of the right glossopharyngeal, vagus and accessory nerves. These three cranial nerves are closely related as they exit from the brainstem but are intimately related as they pass through the jugular foramen. The lesion is most likely to be situated at that level.

The choice of imaging procedure would be influenced by the suspected pathology. If bone erosion around the jugular foramen is suspected, then computerised tomography with bony windows of the skull base would be preferred to bone scanning. Magnetic resonance imaging would be most valuable in delineating the nature of the pathological process supplemented, if the lesion was suspected to be vascular, by either magnetic resonance angiography or formal angiography.

There is a recognised association between AIDS and primary central nervous system lymphoma. Most of these tumours (which tend to be multiple) are found within the brain parenchyma, typically in the periventricular regions but extra-axial occurrence is recognised and is the likeliest cause of this patient's jugular foramen syndrome.

Primary central nervous system lymphoma, in the absence of AIDS, is usually responsive, at least initially, to a combination of irradiation and corticosteroid therapy. In AIDS patients the response is poor and the patient is unlikely to survive more than 6 months.

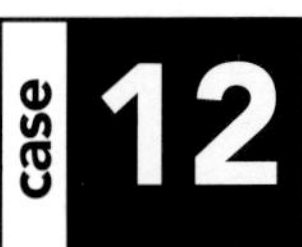

DIFFERENTIAL DIAGNOSIS

1. Pyloric stenosis (infantile hypertrophic pyloric stenosis)
2. Gastro-oesophageal reflux

DISCUSSION

Pyloric stenosis is a relatively common surgical diagnosis in the young infant in the first half of the first year. It can be diagnosed entirely clinically. The laboratory tests are really to ascertain the degree of biochemical derangement so that it can be corrected before surgery and ensure a safer anaesthetic during surgery.

The biochemistry demonstrates a picture of a partially compensated hypochloraemic alkalosis (low chloride, elevated pH and bicarbonate with a compensatory rise in pCO_2 and fall in potassium) and moderate dehydration (raised urea). This is a result of vomiting stomach contents (hydrogen and chloride ions) and the compensatory homeostatic mechanisms.

The baby needs an immediate bolus of 20 ml/kg of normal (0.9%) saline to resuscitate the circulation (repeated if necessary), in addition to maintenance fluids (e.g. 120 ml/kg/day) of 4% dextrose and 0.18% (isotonic) with maintenance potassium added. After a nasogastric tube is passed, normal saline with added potassium needs to be given, in addition to the maintenance fluids, on a millilitre for millilitre basis after each hourly nasogastric aspirate is measured.

Once the biochemistry is normal (usually within 24–48 h) then a pyloromyotomy (Ramstedt's) operation is carried out. The infant is normally back on full enteral feeds within 24–36 h and then discharged home completely well.

case 13

DIFFERENTIAL DIAGNOSIS

1. Right-sided heart failure
2. Hypoproteineamic states, for example, chronic liver disease, nephrotic syndrome or protein-losing enteropathy
3. Inferior vena cava obstruction
4. Unilateral oedema: think of local causes, for example, deep venous thrombosis, soft tissue or bony injury, ruptured Baker's cyst or cellulitis

DISCUSSION

The presenting complaint of this patient is oedema. The causes of bilateral pedal oedema are distinct from unilateral oedema. The other complaints are of fatigue and pruritus. The history also details insulin-dependent diabetes and a positive family history of ischaemic heart disease. The patient presumably also suffers from ischaemic heart disease because she uses sublingual nitrates and has an irregularly irregular pulse treated with digoxin (presumably atrial fibrillation). From the history, therefore, the most likely cause would be oedema secondary to congestive cardiac failure. Chronic liver disease is the other differential diagnosis because of the symptoms of fatigue and pruritus.

The striking abnormalities on clinical examination are white nails (leukonychia), jaundice, xanthelasmata and bilateral pedal oedema. The pansystolic murmur (which is compatible with mitral regurgitation) and atrial fibrillation are presumably secondary to ischaemic heart disease that is coincidental. The cause of this patient's ischaemic heart disease is probably diabetes.

Leukonychia is a clinical sign indicative of a hypoproteineamic state. Any hypoproteinaemic state may lead to leukonychia and causes involve impaired protein synthesis (chronic liver disease) or a protein-losing state (protein-losing enteropathy or nephrotic syndrome). Jaundice indicates here that the cause is due to hepatic decompensation. Fatigue is a common presenting symptom in chronic liver disease. A middle-aged or elderly lady presenting with jaundice, xanthelesmata, pruritus and fatigue should alert the clinician to the most likely diagnosis of primary biliary cirrhosis. The presence of a palpable spleen indicates portal hypertension.

Xanthelesmata or xanthomas occur in hyperlipidaemic states. There are a number of hereditary hyperlipidaemic states that are often associated with cardiac morbidity. The other common cause for xanthelesmata or xanthomata is cholestatic liver disease, most commonly primary biliary cirrhosis.

Primary biliary cirrhosis occurs most commonly in middle-aged women and often presents with pruritus without jaundice. Fatigue is also a common complaint. The striking histological abnormality is bile duct destruction which has been related to immunological disturbance (the mitochondrial antibody M2 is specific for primary biliary cirrhosis). Cirrhosis with jaundice occurs usually within 2.5 years of the onset of pruritus. Skin xanthomas are a common finding and skin hyperpigmentation can be a feature. Osteoporosis and portal hypertension (leading to bleeding oesophageal varices) may present problems. Liver function tests are cholestatic: raised alkaline phosphatase and gamma-glutamyl transferase, with or without an increase in bilirubin. Diagnosis is by liver biopsy. Treatment used is ursodeoxycholic acid and hepatic transplantation.

case 14

DIFFERENTIAL DIAGNOSIS

1. Acute left heart failure
   – Acute aortic insufficiency
   – Mitral insufficiency
2. Atypical pneumonia
3. Myocarditis
4. Cardiomyopathy
5. Hypertension
6. Acute renal failure
7. Silent myocardial infarction

DISCUSSION

The most likely diagnosis after taking the history is acute left heart failure (note the paroxysmal nocturnal dyspnoea) but an atypical pneumonia cannot be excluded at this stage. Possible causes of acute left heart failure include acute aortic or mitral insufficiency, either because of mechanical disruption of a congenitally abnormal valve or because of damage from endocarditis. In patients with Marfan's syndrome, dissecting aneurysm of the descending aorta can also cause an acute aortic reflux. Other possible causes include a myocarditis or cardiomyopathy, undiagnosed hypertension, acute renal failure or silent myocardial infarction. The rapid rate of progression is important, it points to a virulent underlying illness and indicates a need for urgent diagnosis, investigation and treatment. The physical signs are of severe aortic regurgitation. Note the early diastolic murmur, the large volume pulse and the wide pulse pressure. The crackles in the lungs are a sign of pulmonary oedema. The possibility of endocarditis should always be considered in a patient with an acute valve lesion. The classic signs of finger clubbing, splinter haemorrhages and enlarged spleen are features of chronic or subacute endocarditis and even then are not found in all cases.

The most important immediate investigation is echocardiography. In this patient it showed severe aortic reflux with a large vegetation on the aortic valve and an aortic root abscess. Blood cultures were negative, possibly because of the short period of (inappropriate) self-medication. The patient required emergency aortic valve surgery. A swab from the abscess eventually grew a streptococcus.

case 15

DIFFERENTIAL DIAGNOSIS

1. Dementia, for example, caused by Alzheimer's disease
2. Pseudodementia caused by depression

DISCUSSION

The clinical picture is that of an early dementia. Characteristic features include the loss of interest in everyday activities, the lessening of skills in habitual tasks, the subtle change of mood and the tendency to ignore or play down these developments. Alzheimer's disease is the likely mechanism. Although there was a history of hypertension, there have been no stroke-like events to suggest multi-infarct dementia. The history of a previous skull fracture is irrelevant except that a correlation exists between Alzheimer's disease and previous head injury.

In the early stages of dementia, the physical examination is likely to be normal, unless a less common pathology than Alzheimer's disease is responsible. A bedside test of intellectual function (e.g. the mini-mental test) is worth performing, as long as it is recognised that some patients in the early stages of dementia will not be identified.

Conventionally, besides routine haematological and biochemical tests, patients with suspected dementia have serum B_{12}, thyroxine and a test for syphilis (VDRL) performed. The chances of vitamin B_{12} deficiency, hypothyroidism or neurosyphilis presenting with a pure dementia syndrome are remote.

The computerised tomography scan, for a 70 year old, is unremarkable. The main value of this or magnetic resonance imaging in the investigation of dementia is to exclude unusual pathologies, for example, a subfrontal meningioma, bilateral subdural haematomas or normal-pressure hydrocephalus. In dementia, there is a poor correlation between the size of the cortical sulci and the presence of intellectual impairment. Some improvement in correlation is found by measuring the diameter of the third ventricle or, with magnetic resonance imaging, by carrying out volumetric studies of the temporal lobes.

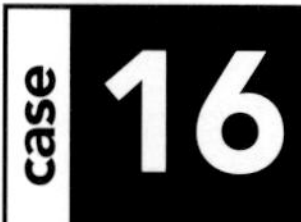

Case 16

DISCUSSION

Urinary tract infections are a common problem in infants and children. This case is an example of how vague or 'atypical' the presentation may be. The younger the child, the more important it is to make the diagnosis and ensure thorough follow-up. Symptoms of urinary tract infections in the very young can be unspecific and therefore hard to detect.

A low threshold to check a urine culture is necessary. This is complicated by the difficulty in obtaining a specimen from infants free of contamination by skin flora from the perineum. Bag specimens need to be collected and interpreted with care. A clean catch is technically problematic but is the gold standard. For some patients a suprapubic aspirate of urine may be the only way to ensure a valid result.

Unrecognised and untreated urinary tract infections are implicated as a cause of nephropathy and renal insufficiency in children. The exact mechanisms of urinary tract infection and renal scarring are still unclear despite extensive studies. It seems likely that the abnormal renal tract with dilated ureters, vesicoureteric reflux, duplex systems and so on are associated with long-term renal damage.

The radiological investigations commonly performed include ultrasound of the entire renal tract to examine the size, shape and position of the kidneys, dilated renal tracts and bladder wall thickness and residual volumes before and after micturition, micturating cystourethrography to examine for vesicoureteric reflux and posterior urethral valves, isotope renal imaging to detect renal scarring (e.g. Di Mercapto Succinic Acid [DMSA] scans) and determine the relative function of each kidney, and other isotope and contrast studies.

This patient had a normal ultrasound, unilateral left-sided reflux on micturating cystourethrography and normal isotope studies. She needs her growth and blood pressure monitoring in the clinic, prophylactic antibiotics at night to prevent infection and a low threshold to check her urine culture if she has any recurring symptoms or unexplained fevers. She is likely to outgrow this problem in the first few years.

All this should be done on the premise to prevent a long-term renal insufficiency that may affect an infant in later life.

case 17

DIFFERENTIAL DIAGNOSIS

1. Watery rhinorrhoea
   - Allergic rhinitis: seasonal
   - Perennial
   - Parasympathetic: dominant vasomotor rhinitis
   - Nasal polyps
   - Adenoidal hypertrophy in children
2. Purulent rhinorrhoea
   - Infective rhinitis or sinusitis
   - Foreign body
3. Bloodstained rhinorrhoea
   - Foreign body
   - Tumour

DISCUSSION

Like most medicine, the history is the key to diagnosis. You need to ask the patient the nature of the discharge, how long it has been present, whether it is constant, whether it is influenced by the time of the year, if there are pets at home, whether he or she is asthmatic or allergic to aspirin, whether there has been any loss of sense of smell, if there has been any change in the shape of his or her nose, whether the blockage is unilateral, bilateral or alternating and whether he or she has used inhaled nasal steroids or had previous sinonasal surgery?

The answers to these questions give a good idea of the nature of the discharge. Usually nasal discharge is associated with a degree of nasal obstruction and once again the history will point to the diagnosis.

case 18

DIFFERENTIAL DIAGNOSIS

1. Benign or malignant oesophageal obstruction
2. An oesophageal motility disorder

Other rarer causes include:

3. Neuromuscular disorders (bulbar palsy, myasthenia gravis)
4. Intrinsic lesions (pharyngeal pouch)
5. Extrinsic pressure (goitre, enlarged left atrium, mediastinal mass or glands)

DISCUSSION

The predominant symptom of the history is dysphagia. This is the principal symptom of oesophageal disease. Like many patients complaining of dysphagia, the patient is able to point to a particular place where the symptom is predominantly felt. However, in clinical practice this is not always helpful as it does not always correspond to the level of obstruction. When faced with a patient complaining of dysphagia, it is important to take a clear history. Ensure that the symptom is true dysphagia because many patients may confuse it with acid reflux, regurgitation or heartburn. Determine the speed of onset, its constancy and whether there is a difference between solids or liquids. Ask about associated symptoms such as weight loss, pain on swallowing (odynophagia) and acid reflux.

Benign oesophageal strictures often occur on a background of significant acid reflux symptoms. Oesophageal carcinoma presents commonly as a rapidly progressive dysphagia (particularly for solids) and is associated with significant weight loss. Oesophageal motility disorders usually present as a more gradual complaint, often occurring intermittently. The disorders that lead to oesophageal motility disorders include achalasia, diffuse oesophageal spasm, nutcracker oesophagus, nonspecific oesophageal motility disorder and systemic sclerosis.

The two most likely causes for this patient's dysphagia is a benign oesophageal stricture or an oesophageal motility disorder. However, a malignancy, although less likely (no weight loss, gradual onset, intermittent) cannot be excluded on history alone. From the history alone, one might suspect a benign oesophageal stricture as a complication of gastro-oesophageal reflux disease (she has a long history of 'indigestion'). One confounding symptom however is the description of symptoms suggestive of Raynaud's phenomenon.

The examination is often unhelpful in elucidating the cause of dysphagia. However, here there are striking abnormalities: skin tethering over the dorsum of the hands and telangiectasiae. These skin signs are very suggestive of systemic sclerosis and this is the diagnosis in this case.

Systemic sclerosis has typical skin appearances. Thickening of the skin characteristically involves the hands, leading to limitation of fine movements and eventually tapering of the fingers called sclerodactly. Facial involvement produces beaking of the nose and limitation of mouth opening. Telangiectasia on the face and hands is common and skin fibrosis surrounding joints may lead to deformities and movement limitation. Up to two-thirds of patients with systemic sclerosis may present initially with Raynaud's phenomenon alone.

Systemic sclerosis is a multi-organ disease. Approximately 90% of cases of systemic sclerosis lead to oesophageal involvement. Typically, there is loss of lower oesophageal sphincter tone and reduced or absent oesophageal peristalsis, leading to a dilated oesophagus at risk of significant acid reflux. Severe cases may result in a benign oesophageal stricture.

Oesophageal involvement by systemic sclerosis is usually made by barium swallow or manometry. Treatment involves a prokinetic in the early stages (which has variable benefit) and acid suppression therapy. Strictures can be dilated endoscopically.

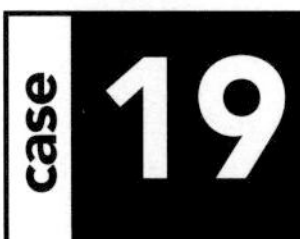

DIFFERENTIAL DIAGNOSIS

1. Lobar pneumonia, probably pneumococcal
2. Underlying bronchiectasis and possibly cystic fibrosis

DISCUSSION

The rapid onset of symptoms in a patient who was previously well strongly suggests an acute lower respiratory tract infection. This is supported by the upper respiratory 'flu symptoms. The pleuritic pain, shortness of breath and purulent sputum with some blood all point to lobar pneumonia. The most likely organism is *Streptococcus pneumoniae* but a primary viral pneumonia is possible. *Staphylococcus aureus* is also common after influenza. Mycoplasma infection is less likely as the onset is slower, with cough as a predominant symptom. The long history of productive cough, although made light of by the patient, is probably significant and suggests some underlying chronic lung disease. Smoking-related chronic bronchitis is the most common cause but this patient is rather young, the smoking is comparatively light and the history goes back to childhood. Only three chest conditions are likely to have their origins in childhood; asthma, bronchiectasis and cystic fibrosis. Asthma is unlikely in this patient with the lack of previous wheeze and breathlessness. Cystic fibrosis only occasionally manifests so late in life, therefore, serious consideration should be given to bronchiectasis. Acquired immunoglobulin deficiency is possible but rare and patients have usually had a succession of acute chest infections before the diagnosis is made.

The examination findings are essentially those of lobar pneumonia. They make mycoplasma and viral infections unlikely and strengthen the possibility of a pneumococcal infection. The herpes infection is a marker for a lower respiratory infection. The crackles at the left base could be no more than some additional acute infection on this side or could just be related to the smoking history. They do, however, support the possibility of some underlying bronchiectasis. It may well be that the combination of influenza and chronic underlying disease has led to the current episode.

The next step will be a chest radiograph to confirm the presence of consolidation together with blood and sputum culture to try and obtain an organism.

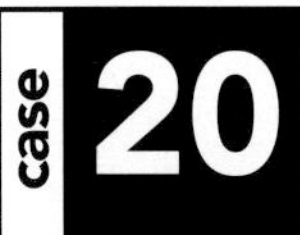

DIFFERENTIAL DIAGNOSIS

1. Microbial infections
2. Immunological reactions
3. Hormones (e.g. thyroxine)
4. Drug reactions
5. Malignancy (e.g. lymphoma)

DISCUSSION

This patient's presenting complaint is fever. The other symptoms of malaise and joint and muscle aches are rather nonspecific. He has a recent history of a probable chest infection. The differential diagnosis from the history would include microbial infections (a partially treated pneumonia, reactivation of old tuberculosis, viral illness) or a drug reaction (recent antibiotic).

The clinical examination confirms a fever. The important finding is a change in the cardiac murmur. When the patient recently attended the hospital outpatient department, there was a murmur suggestive of mitral regurgitation (quiet first heart sound, pansystolic murmur maximal at the apex and radiating to the axilla). Currently, the murmur is ejection systolic at the left sternal edge. The causes of such a murmur are aortic flow, aortic sclerosis or stenosis, pulmonary stenosis or left outflow tract obstruction. Rather than finding clinical signs suggestive of a respiratory infection (dull percussion note, coarse inspiratory crepitations, increased vocal resonance, bronchial breathing), the current signs indicate heart failure (raised jugular venous pressure and bilateral fine basal inspiratory crepitations).

The combination of a fever, changing heart murmur and cardiac failure is in keeping with a diagnosis of infective endocarditis.

Infective endocarditis is an infection of the endocardium. It is an uncommon cause of a fever. It can present acutely or subacutely. Infection occurs commonly on rheumatic, congenitally abnormal or prosthetic valves. The most common organisms are *Streptococcus viridans, Streptococcus faecalis* and *Staphylococcus aureus.*

There are a large number of clinical findings associated with infective endocarditis. These include malaise, pyrexia, heart murmurs or failure, microscopic haematuria, splenomegaly, arthralgia, skin lesions (petechiae, Osler's nodes, splinter haemorrhages, Janeway lesions), clubbing, Roth spots and cerebral emboli or mycotic aneurysms.

A high index of suspicion for infective endocarditis

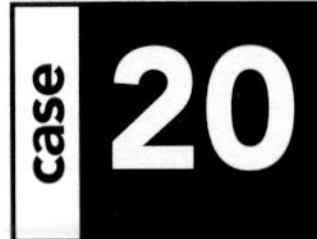

is warranted in patients with prosthetic heart valves and a fever. Confirmation of the diagnosis is by blood cultures (often at least six sets) and echocardiography to visualise vegetations. Treatment is guided by sensitivities of blood cultures. Initial treatment is usually a combination of a penicillin and gentamicin which is continued for 6 weeks.

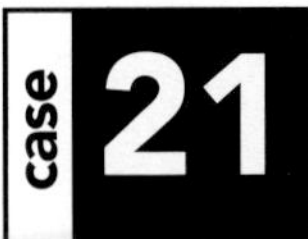

DIFFERENTIAL DIAGNOSIS

1. Lateral medullary syndrome
2. Vertebral artery dissection
3. Vertebral artery embolism
4. Vertebral artery thrombosis

DISCUSSION

The clinical picture of a left Horner's syndrome, left trigeminal sensory loss, left palatal palsy, left-sided cerebellar signs and contralateral spino-thalamic loss is characteristic of the lateral medullary syndrome (Wallenberg's syndrome). Typical symptomatology of this condition includes intense vertigo and intractable hiccoughs.

Contrary to popular teaching, the primary pathology lies not in the posterior inferior cerebellar artery but in the parent vertebral artery. The condition is generally seen in older people. The pathology is usually in-situ occlusion of the vertebral artery by thrombus associated with arteriosclerosis. Occasionally, embolism of the vertebral artery from a proximal source, for example, the heart, is responsible. Clearly, atheroma is unlikely here; the patient suffered a neck injury the day before and, associated with his symptoms, he had complained of an intense pain behind the left ear. Vertebral artery dissection is the diagnosis of choice. Although it may occur spontaneously, classically it follows a neck injury or over-vigorous neck manipulation. The time between trauma and the onset of symptoms may be hours, as in this case, or several weeks.

There are a number of alternative investigations. Doppler studies of the neck arteries should show dampened flow in the relevant vertebral artery with normal flow contralaterally. Magnetic resonance imaging (MRI) can detect a thrombus associated with the dissection by an abnormal signal from the relevant vessel. Magnetic resonance angiography (MRA) is probably not sufficiently sensitive to unequivocally declare the diagnosis but will certainly establish the presence of abnormal flow. Formal angiography usually shows pathognomonic features, particularly a tapering occlusion or a long segment narrowing (string sign) of the affected vessel

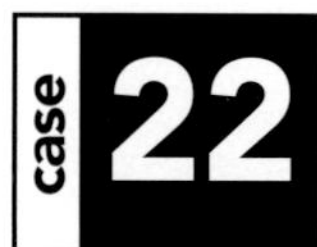

DIFFERENTIAL DIAGNOSIS

1. Bacterial meningitis
2. Encephalitis
3. First febrile convulsion with upper respiratory infection

DISCUSSION

This girl is critically ill and needs prompt investigation and treatment. As with all critically ill patients, attention should be given to the 'ABC' of resuscitation: **A**irway first, then **B**reathing and only then **C**irculation. A drowsy patient such as this may require intubation and ventilation.

Once the **ABC** has been addressed, intravascular access should be gained and blood samples sent for cultures, glucose, blood count and electrolytes.

As bacterial meningitis is very likely and the baby is critically ill, current opinion suggests that lumbar puncture is best deferred until she is clinically more stable. There is evidence that dexamethasone given intravenously before, or at the same time as, antibiotics decreases some of the long-term morbidity of bacterial meningitis (e.g. sensorineural deafness).

This girl should receive dexamethasone intravenously, followed by a powerful broad spectrum antibiotic that will cover the likely pathogens (i.e. a fourth generation cephalosporin such as ceftriaxone) and an antiviral drug (acyclovir). If the cerebrospinal fluid findings suggest an encephalitis or viral meningitis, herpes simplex virus can be safely treated before the diagnosis is suspected or confirmed.

This girl required 24 h of mechanical ventilation on intensive care and a cranial computerised tomography scan did not show signs of critical cerebral oedema. A lumbar puncture was performed and showed the following results:

Cerebrospinal fluid:	
White blood cell count	**127 (75% neutrophils)**
Red blood cell count	**47 per mm^3**
Protein	**1.9 g/l**
Glucose	**2.4 mmol/l**
Gram stain	**No organisms seen**
Latex antigen tests	**Positive for *Streptococcus pneumoniae***
Plasma	**Glucose 6.9 mmol/l**

The absence of Gram-positive cocci on Gram staining reflects the delay in performing the lumbar puncture in the face of parenteral antibiotics. Cerebrospinal antigen tests and polymerase chain reaction assays for the bacterial genome can determine an accurate diagnosis. It is worth remembering that blood cultures are positive in over two-thirds of patients with meningitis. This girl's blood cultures were also positive for *Streptococcus pneumoniae*.

The child was treated for 14 days with parenteral antibiotics before discharge. She remained unsteady and withdrawn during the first 10 days after leaving hospital but was clearly making progress.

The outpatient review, including an audiogram, demonstrated a profound unilateral sensorineural hearing loss in the left ear and high frequency hearing loss in the right ear. She now requires bilateral hearing aids.

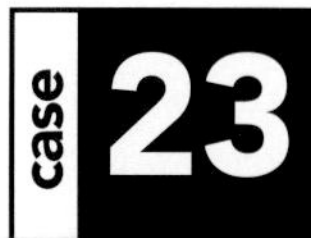

DIFFERENTIAL DIAGNOSIS

1. Infected lymph node
2. Malignant lymph node
3. Branchial cyst

DISCUSSION

Enlarged lymph nodes in the neck are most commonly infective in origin. The focus of infection is usually in the upper aerodigestive tract but may arise from the skin of the scalp, face and neck.

However, in older patients malignancy must be excluded. Primary malignancies of the head and neck spread preferentially to cervical nodes. The history must therefore seek symptoms related to the mouth and throat, including pain and swallowing. Smoking and alcohol intake, particularly in combination, are potent aetiological factors in these malignancies. Poor oral and dental hygiene is also a useful pointer. The examination must include all possible primary sites and must not focus only on the node in the neck.

Further investigations will include a chest radiograph because there may be synchronous chest disease (especially bearing in mind the aetiological factors mentioned) or secondary spread. A biopsy of the primary lesion together with fine needle aspiration cytology of the neck mass is mandatory before any decision is taken on the definitive treatment of the neck mass.

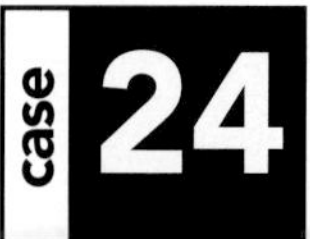

DIFFERENTIAL DIAGNOSIS

1. Prehepatic (haemolysis)
2. Hepatic (Gilberts, hepatitis, cirrhosis)
3. Cholestasis (drugs, biliary obstruction)

DISCUSSION

The presenting complaint is jaundice. When taking a history from a patient with jaundice there are a number of questions that need to be asked such as recent travel, alcohol and drug misuse, previous blood transfusions, stool and urine colour change, contact illnesses, recent medications, family history, presence of pruritus and sexual orientation. This valuable information may aid the clinician in forming a diagnosis.

The relevant features in this man's history include a past blood transfusion, recent ingestion of erythromycin and recent increased alcohol intake after a marital breakdown (suspect drug overdose especially paracetamol). The differential from the history could therefore justifiably be an alcohol-related liver disease, viral hepatitis, drug reaction or paracetamol overdose.

A worrying clinical finding in a patient with jaundice is confusion. There are a number of possible causes of confusion in a patient with jaundice. The agitation and fine tremor in this patient suggests alcohol withdrawal. Hepatic encephalopathy is a further important cause. The tremor of hepatic encephalopathy is a coarse involuntary flap best demonstrated with the patient's arms outstretched and the hands extended at the wrist and metacarpophalangeal joints. Confusion caused by Wernicke–Korsakoff syndrome classically involves an encephalopathy accompanied by ophthalmoplegia, nystagmus and ataxia. Confusion can also be caused by unrelated general causes in a jaundiced patient for example, infection.

The main clinical findings in this patient are jaundice, confusion, fine tremor, absence of stigmata of chronic liver disease, mild fever, hepatomegaly and a hepatic bruit. There are only a small number of causes for a hepatic bruit namely, alcoholic hepatitis, hepatocellular carcinoma and acute viral hepatitis. It is for this reason that auscultation to detect a bruit can be very helpful in patients with hepatomegaly or jaundice. The acute presentation and lack of signs of chronic liver disease would be against hepatocellular carcinoma. There is no history of recent exposure for viral hepatitis. The combination of a recent history of increased alcohol intake,

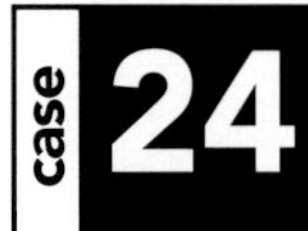

signs suggestive of alcohol withdrawal and a hepatic bruit would be most in keeping with a diagnosis of alcoholic hepatitis.

An important finding when examining a patient with jaundice is the presence or absence of stigmata of chronic liver disease. These include clubbing, white nails, Dupuyteron's contracture, palmar erythema, spider naevi, gynaecomastia, splenomegaly, dilated abdominal veins, ascites, testicular atrophy, parotid swelling and fetor hepatis.

Alcoholic hepatitis occurs in its most severe case when a patient has been drinking particularly heavily and not eating. The episode may be precipitated by a general illness, for example, infection. There may be tender enlarged hepatomegaly. Complications such as hepatic decompensation, hepatorenal syndrome or bleeding oesophageal varices may occur. Liver function tests show raised liver transaminases and bilirubin. Liver biopsy is diagnostic. Mortality rate can be up to 50%. Treatment is good nutritional care and careful attention to complications. Patients who are selected according to the calculation of an arithmetic discriminant factor (calculated by prothrombin time and bilirubin) may benefit from corticosteroids if sepsis, viral hepatitis and gastrointestinal bleeding are not concurrent problems.

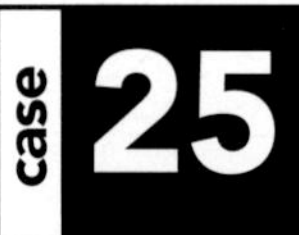

DIFFERENTIAL DIAGNOSIS

1. Disc disease
2. Intrinsic cord tumour
3. Extra-axial tumour

DISCUSSION

The history is strongly suggestive of a degenerative process affecting the neck. The previous history suggests a radicular disturbance in the upper limbs with pain radiating to the arm and sensory symptoms in the hand. Coupled with these symptoms were problems in the lower limbs which suggested the likelihood of an upper motor neuron syndrome. This combination, which incorporated both motor and sensory features, suggests a diagnosis of cervical spondylosis with both radicular and myelopathic components.

The history and physical findings indicate the presence of fasciculation and weakness in right triceps. Triceps is supplied by the sixth and seventh cervical roots. There is equivocal weakness of the small hand muscles on the right but from the other information given this is likely to represent the myelopathic rather than the radicular component of the problem. The only sensory symptom is paraesthesiae in the right index finger with, on examination, some blunting of cutaneous sensation in the same digit. The index finger is supplied by the sixth cervical root. The patient has inversion of the right biceps and supinator reflexes. The finger flexion that accompanied these reflexes was mirrored by the finding of brisk finger jerks. The biceps and supinator reflexes are supplied by cervical segments five and six, the finger jerks by segment eight. An inverted biceps or supinator reflex implies interruption of the reflex arc at that level, with spread to a lower segmental level, the consequence of the spindles in muscles supplied by that lower level being primed by the presence of a myelopathy affecting the cord from the C5/C6 segment down.

The alternative investigations are computerised tomography, myelography or magnetic resonance imaging (MRI) of the cervical spine. MRI is noninvasive and is the preferred technique.

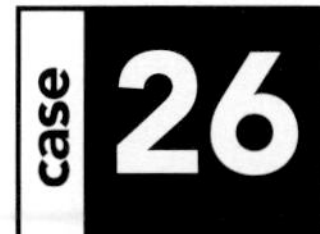

DIFFERENTIAL DIAGNOSIS

1. Primary skin conditions (including eczema, urticaria, insect bites, scabies)
2. Systemic disorders (including cholestasis, lymphoma, uraemia, drugs, hyperthyroidism, polycythaemia rubra vera, diabetes, carcinoid syndrome)

DISCUSSION

Often a clear history with attention to associated features can be useful when a patient presents with pruritus. Ascertaining whether the symptom stems from a primary skin complaint or a more generalised systemic disorder is the first step. Ask about the location of the pruritus, whether there is recent drug ingestion, travel, any contact illness or insect bites. Careful examination of the skin for a rash or discharge is important. Generalised symptoms should be noted.

This patient's pruritus is generalised and without a rash. One would suspect a systemic illness. There has been no recent change in his medication. He is not jaundiced and has no other features for carcinoid syndrome. The differential from the history would include hyperthyroidism, lymphoma, uraemia or polycythaemia rubra vera.

The clinical examination confirms a euthyroid state. There is hepatosplenomegaly without lymphadenopathy. The plethora suggests polycythaemia rubra vera. The description of the pruritus (worse after a hot bath) is typical for polycythaemia rubra vera.

Polycythaemia is caused by a raised red cell volume that is reflected in a high haemoglobin level. The causes of polycythaemia include primary polycythaemia rubra vera, secondary to hypoxia (lung disease, high altitude, heavy smoking), primary polycythaemia rubra vera secondary to raised erythropoeitin (renal disease or carcinoma) and 'relative' causes (stress, dehydration).

Polycythaemia rubra vera often presents in later years with nonspecific symptoms. It is an uncommon cause of pruritus. There is a tendency to angina, claudication and hypertension. Clinical examination often reveals plethora, conjunctival infection, dusky colouration of the tongue and hepatosplenomegaly. Examination of the fundi indicates venous engorgement with 'sausage' shaped vessels. Investigations will reveal a raised haemoglobin and red cell volume with normal blood gases and a raised red cell mass. Bone marrow shows erythroid hyperplasia. Treatment is initially by venesection and chemotherapy.

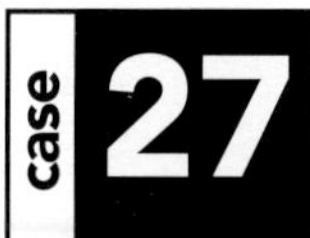

DIFFERENTIAL DIAGNOSIS

1. Thyroglossal cyst
2. Lymph node
3. Lipoma

DISCUSSION

The key to diagnosis here is the fact that this is a midline swelling that moves with protrusion of the tongue; lymph nodes are infrequently in the midline and they do not move with tongue protrusion. Subcutaneous lesions also do not move and may be attached to the overlying skin. Thyroglossal cysts are typically in the midline but may be 'off centre'.

If the possibility of lymphadenopathy arises, other lymph node sites, for example, the axillae and groins, should be examined to exclude a generalised disease process.

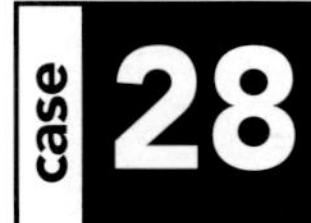

DIFFERENTIAL DIAGNOSIS

1. Atrial fibrillation
2. Atrial flutter
3. Mitral valve disease
4. Atrial septal defect
5. Hyperthyroidism
6. Alcohol misuse

DISCUSSION

Common causes of palpitation can be divided into the intermittent and the continuous. The most common causes of continuous palpitation are atrial fibrillation and atrial flutter. Ectopic beats may be frequent but seldom start suddenly and continue without intermission. The persistent tachycardia of untreated atrial fibrillation can cause heart failure. Although many cases of atrial fibrillation have no detectable cause and are called lone atrial fibrillation, this diagnosis should never be accepted without a search for predisposing factors. These include mitral valve disease, congenital heart disease in the form of an atrial septal defect, an overactive thyroid gland or alcohol misuse. In this patient, echocardiography confirmed a moderately-sized atrial septal defect (note split second heart sound) but this diagnosis had not really been expected. She also had biochemical evidence of an overactive thyroid and raised liver enzymes compatible with increased alcohol consumption. Real cases are not always straightforward.

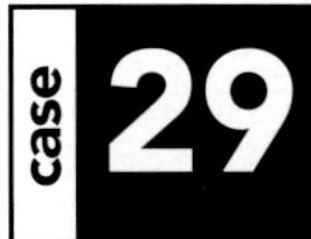

DIFFERENTIAL DIAGNOSIS

1. Lung cancer
2. Tuberculosis

DISCUSSION

Lung cancer and tuberculosis are the most important causes to consider in this patient. The most common cause of haemoptysis, however, is acute infection either with or without underlying structural disease such as chronic bronchitis or bronchiectasis. The other important common cause is pulmonary embolism. Rarer causes are bronchial adenoma, idiopathic pulmonary haemosiderosis, mitral stenosis and clotting disorders.

The social background is important in this patient. The heavy and prolonged history of smoking is important for the diagnosis of lung cancer because the disease is rare in life-long nonsmokers. Remember, however, that patients often stop smoking weeks or months before the diagnosis is made. They will then report themselves as nonsmokers. Despite his denial, there is circumstantial evidence of alcohol abuse. This may be important in the development of tuberculosis, probably by reducing resistance to infection. Exposure to infectious people in bars is also important. Behind all this there is probably significant clinical depression relating to the death of his wife; this may need to be addressed separately.

The episode in 1945 needs to be explored. To be invalided out of the army suggests a prolonged illness. As a young man the most likely diagnosis must be tuberculosis. At that time there was no effective pharmacological treatment; prolonged rest being the only management. In many patients the disease could be arrested but not necessarily cured. Viable bacteria could remain and later re-activate the disease. The reasons for re-activation are rarely explicit but probably involve some diminution in immune defence as could occur with advancing age or alcohol abuse.

The examination is not very helpful apart from directing attention to the left upper chest. The mild fever could be due to tuberculosis or infection associated with lung cancer or to the cancer itself. The signs suggest some collapse in the left chest but both tuberculosis and lung cancer could cause this. If the finding of clubbing is confirmed, then lung cancer is very probable; only extensive prolonged tuberculosis is associated with clubbing.

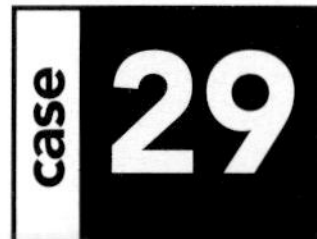

A careful search should be made for supraclavicular lymph nodes. If found, these are much more likely to be caused by secondary cancer than by tuberculosis.

The next steps should be a chest radiograph and examination of the sputum for tuberculosis and malignant cells. The radiograph may be very suggestive of either but of course cannot be diagnostic. Sputum examination may show tuberculous bacilli on direct smear but if negative, it may be necessary to wait for results of culture. A bronchoscopy may visualise a tumour and a biopsy may be possible. It is important to remember that both diseases can occur together; cancer can arise in an old tuberculous scar and a new cancer can re-activate old tubercular disease.

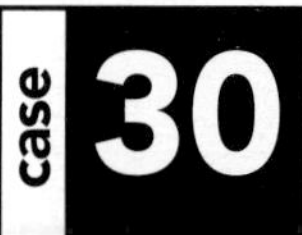

DIFFERENTIAL DIAGNOSIS

1. Vasovagal faint
2. Arrhythmia
   - Ventricular tachycardia
   - Ventricular fibrillation
3. Hypertrophic cardiomyopathy
4. Myocarditis
5. Wolff–Parkinson–White syndrome
6. Anomalous coronary artery
7. Aortic stenosis

DISCUSSION

The most common cause of syncope in a young person is a simple vasovagal faint. However, the circumstances here are very unusual for a faint and syncope that is precipitated by, or follows, exertion must be taken seriously. There is nothing to suggest epilepsy, and by far the most likely cause is cardiovascular. Possible causes include an arrhythmia, usually ventricular tachycardia or fibrillation; this in turn may be due to hypertrophic cardiomyopathy, myocarditis, Wolff–Parkinson–White syndrome or an anomalous coronary artery. Nonarrhythmic, effort-related syncope can also occur in severe aortic stenosis or hypertrophic cardiomyopathy. By definition, patients with syncope are unable to give a very clear account of what happened, so information from witnesses is always helpful.

The findings on physical examination are strongly suggestive of hypertrophic cardiomyopathy. The double apex beat is the result of atrial hypertrophy in response to a hypertrophied and stiff left ventricle; hence also the fourth heart sound. The systolic murmur is caused by left ventricular outflow obstruction which gets worse when venous return is diminished, for example, immediately after exercise. The condition is inherited by an autosomal dominant gene and you would expect to find it in 50% of the siblings of an affected patient. However, the new mutation rate is high and this may account for the fairly frequent patient with no known family history.

The diagnosis of hypertrophic cardiomyopathy was confirmed by echocardiography. Supervised exercise testing precipitated a ventricular arrhythmia that fortunately was self-terminating. He was eventually treated with a ß-blocker and an implanted defibrillator. His younger brother was screened and found to be free of the condition.

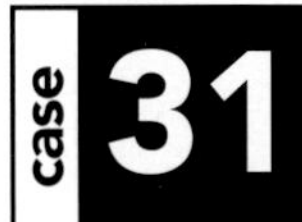

case 31

DIFFERENTIAL DIAGNOSIS

1. Cryptogenic fibrosing alveolitis
2. Asbestosis

DISCUSSION

The history is of progressive shortness of breath over a few weeks. The most likely causes are chronic airflow limitation, alveolitis, left ventricular failure, pleural effusion and anaemia. The history is a little short for chronic airflow limitation and the absence of wheeze or of any variability in the symptoms is also against the diagnosis. The chronic productive cough and the history of smoking are suggestive of an airway problem but could be coincidental. The treatment with diuretics suggests that the referring practitioner considered left ventricular failure but the failure to respond even in part suggests an alternative diagnosis. Furthermore, there are no other features in the history to suggest cardiac dyspnoea, neither is there a history of cardiac disease. A pleural effusion or anaemia is possible and should be easily confirmed or excluded on examination.

The social history is intriguing. A worker in the construction industry has almost inevitably been exposed to asbestos in the past even if he has not handled it himself. Asbestosis cannot at this stage be excluded. Protein antigens derived from budgerigars are a cause of extrinsic allergic alveolitis. The drug history is important because a number can cause lung fibrosis; the most common are amiodarone and many anticancer drugs.

The examination makes a cardiac cause even less likely and also helps to exclude anaemia and a pleural effusion for which a deviated trachea, localised dullness and reduced breath sounds would be expected. The clubbing, if confirmed, would make extrinsic allergic alveolitis unlikely but strengthens the case for asbestosis and cryptogenic fibrosing alveolitis. The dullness at both lung bases could be caused by bilateral effusions but is more likely to be caused by raised diaphragms from loss of lung volume. The crackles are suggestive of a problem at the alveolar level and their presence helps to exclude sarcoidosis which is notable for the absence of lung signs even when the chest radiograph is markedly abnormal. Their presence at the lung bases would be unusual in extrinsic allergic alveolitis when they are mainly in the mid or upper zones.

The next step will be to obtain a chest radiograph and pulmonary function tests.

case 32

DIFFERENTIAL DIAGNOSIS

1. All gastrointestinal disorders
2. Many malignancies
3. Thyrotoxicosis
4. Diabetes mellitus
5. Psychiatric disorders, for example, anorexia nervosa
6. Any severe illness

DISCUSSION

There are many causes of weight loss. It is helpful in clinical practice to have weight loss documented objectively. Ask about appetite, over what timespan the weight has been lost, dietary intake and any other symptoms.

This patient's weight loss has been chronic and associated with epigastric pain. There appears to be a clear relation between the pain and meals. Under normal circumstances, the differential diagnosis of recurrent epigastric pain includes peptic ulceration, pancreatic disease, nonulcer dyspepsia, gallstones (typically right hypochondrium), aortic aneurysm and colonic pathology. Epigastric pain exacerbated by meals normally indicates peptic ulceration, pancreatitis or mesenteric angina.

From the history alone, a differential diagnosis for this patient's weight loss is peptic ulceration, gastric malignancy or pancreatic disease.

The clinical examination substantiates weight loss and epigastric tenderness. The significant finding is a pale stool suggestive of steatorrhoea. The combination of epigastric pain exacerbated by meals, weight loss, polyuria and steatorrhoea suggests pancreatic disease. The chronicity of her symptoms infer the diagnosis of chronic pancreatitis. A pancreatic neoplasm should be excluded.

The main causes of chronic pancreatitis are alcohol (most common), idiopathic and hyperlipidaemia. The enjoyment of sherry in the afternoon hints at the cause in this patient. The development of diabetes is common and again this is suggested in this patient because of the polyuria. Investigation involves combination of ultrasonography, computerised tomography and endoscopic retrograde cholangiopancreatography. Pancreatic neoplasia needs exclusion. Assessment for diabetes is necessary. Treatment involves abstention from alcohol in alcoholic pancreatitis. Pain control can present a difficult problem. Steatorrhoea is treated with pancreatic supplements.

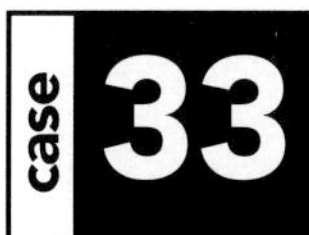

DIFFERENTIAL DIAGNOSIS

1. Gout
2. Septic arthritis
3. Rheumatoid arthritis

DISCUSSION

Gout is by far the most likely diagnosis. The history of a previous attack (albeit in an unusual joint to be affected), the acuteness of the onset and the striking focal changes are all particularly suggestive. Hypertension is associated with gout, as is obesity. Excess alcohol consumption is known to be associated with hyperuricaemia. The rapid response to a nonsteroidal anti-inflammatory drug does not suggest either a septic arthritis or acute rheumatoid arthritis. A low grade fever and a slightly elevated white cell count are both recognised with an acute attack of gout. An acute attack of gout can be triggered, in a susceptible individual, by the use of a thiazide diuretic.

The casualty officer ordered a urate level, which was reported as 8.8 mg/dl. He had a useful discussion with a rheumatology consultant about the desirability of joint aspiration in such cases. The rheumatologist pointed out that joint aspiration was the only certain way to rule out septic arthritis in such cases at the initial presentation, although he admitted that he also might have managed the patient in the same way. In the case of gout, joint aspiration reveals urate crystals. Although the leukocyte count is elevated, the joint fluid is sterile.

The patient should be advised to lose weight, reduce his alcohol intake and avoid diuretic therapy. Once the acute attack has subsided completely, the patient should be prescribed allupurinol covered initially by prophylactic doses of colchicine.

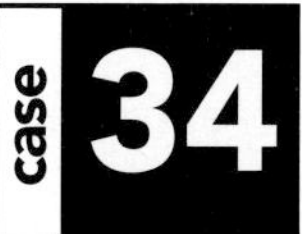

DIFFERENTIAL DIAGNOSIS

1. Heart failure caused by ischaemic heart disease
2. Tuberculous peritonitis suggested by the patient's ethnic origin
3. Malignancy suggested by weight loss
4. Cirrhosis of the liver
5. Nephrotic syndrome

DISCUSSION

There are three possible causes of ascites in this patient that should be considered: heart failure, tuberculous peritonitis and malignancy.

Firstly, heart failure, with a history of a myocardial infarction and ingestion of atenolol (a negatively inotropic agent), should be considered. However, the absence of physical findings of tachycardia, gallop rhythm, elevated jugular venous pressure, basal crackles and peripheral oedema excludes this diagnosis. The increasing difficulty in breathing results from elevation of the diaphragm because of the ascites.

The absence of peripheral oedema suggests that ascites in this patient is not caused by a transudate (ascitic protein content <30 g/l) but is caused by an exudate (ascitic protein content >30 g/l). Causes of transudate include cirrhosis of liver, heart failure, nephrotic syndrome, protein-losing enteropathy, constrictive pericarditis, Meig's syndrome and bacterial veno-occlusive disease. Causes of exudate include fungal or tuberculous peritoneal infection, primary or secondary malignancy and myeloproliferative or lymphoproliferative disease. The absence of peripheral oedema suggests that the ascites results from an intra-abdominal cause.

Tuberculous peritonitis causing ascites is unlikely in the absence of evidence of past or present pulmonary tuberculosis.

In this patient an intra-abdominal malignancy from either an ovarian, pancreatic or gastrointestinal primary, is the most likely diagnosis. An ascitic tap with cytology and abdominal imaging would help confirm the diagnosis.

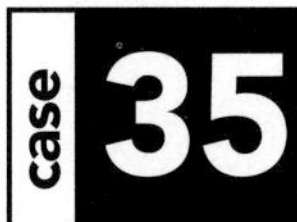

DIFFERENTIAL DIAGNOSIS

1. Peripheral nerve entrapment
2. Cervical radiculopathy
3. Cerebrovascular accident

DISCUSSION

The distribution of muscle weakness and the sensory findings are entirely consistent with a right ulnar nerve lesion. The overwhelming majority of ulnar nerve lesions occur at the elbow. Most of these arise at the level of the ulnar groove or from compression by the aponeurosis of flexor carpi ulnaris within the cubital tunnel. Distal ulnar nerve lesions, either at the wrist or affecting the deep branch of the nerve within the palm, are much rarer.

Ideally, to establish on clinical grounds that an ulnar nerve lesion is at the elbow, you need to demonstrate weakness in all the muscles innervated by the nerve below that level. This would include, therefore, flexor carpi ulnaris and flexor digitorum profundus to the fourth and fifth digits. In addition, you would hope to find a positive Tinel's sign at the elbow, with percussion at that site producing a shower of paraesthesiae in the distal cutaneous distribution of the nerve. In practice, many ulnar nerve lesions at the elbow spare the long flexors and many patients with such lesions have a negative Tinel's sign, whereas many normal individuals without signs of an ulnar paresis will have a positive sign.

Nerve conduction studies are required to establish firmly the diagnosis. There may be an absent or depressed ulnar nerve sensory action potential but the most sensitive techniques are either the demonstration of slowing of motor conduction across the elbow or a prolonged latency to flexor carpi ulnaris after stimulation of the nerve above the medial epicondyle.

The ulnar nerve has almost certainly been damaged at the elbow while the patient has been bedbound and receiving intravenous fluids into that arm. Perhaps further medico-legal action is in the offing!

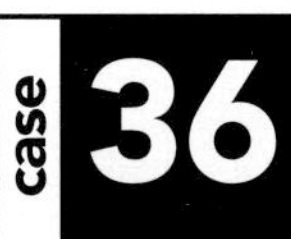

DIFFERENTIAL DIAGNOSIS

1. Asthma (first presentation)
2. Respiratory tract infection
3. Pertussis or a parapertussis infection

DISCUSSION

A lymphocytosis is often seen inpertussis or whooping cough. The boy is started on a course of clarithromycin. His parents are told that the cough will take weeks or months to subside and that the severity of the paroxysms should subside with time. The asthma treatment is discontinued and his parents are urged to stop smoking (or at the very least, to not smoke in the home) because passive smoking is likely to trigger coughing.

Pertussis is a highly infectious respiratory illness that carries with it a mortality in infants in the first 6 months and morbidity in older infants and children. UK vaccination programmes started in the 1950s drastically reduced the prevalence of pertussis but when there were doubts about vaccine safety in the 1970s, immunisation uptake fell and there were more epidemics.

Vaccination is strongly recommended as a way of preventing infection. Doubts about vaccine safety have been unproven despite extensive studies and the previously 'slack' contra-indications to the vaccination have been tightened. The UK currently achieves a 95% coverage by the age of 2 years.

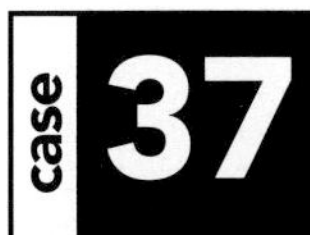

DIFFERENTIAL DIAGNOSIS

1. Laryngeal carcinoma
2. Benign laryngeal tumour or polyp
3. Chronic laryngitis

DISCUSSION

Any patient with a hoarse voice that persists for longer than 4 weeks, should have his or her larynx inspected. The presumptive diagnosis of laryngitis should only follow an event that could have acted as a precipitant, for example, respiratory tract infection, excessive shouting or inhalation of noxious fumes or gases. Any adult over the age of 25 years (more commonly over 40 years old) who develops hoarseness for no apparent reason must be presumed to have a laryngeal malignancy until otherwise proven. Malignancy of the upper aerodigestive tract is uncommon in nonsmokers but may occur in passive smokers. The history of excessive voice usage can be distracting but the fact that the patient was a heavy smoker makes the diagnosis of malignancy more likely.

When examining these patients it is important to look for other lesions (synchronous primaries) throughout the upper aerodigestive tract because the carcinogen (cigarette smoke) may induce malignancy at more than one site in a susceptible field of mucosa.

The most common site of secondary spread from an upper aerodigestive tract malignancy is to the lymph nodes of the neck. The prognosis in these patients is significantly affected by the extent of spread to the neck. Although distant metastases (mainly to the lungs) usually occur late in the disease, they must be excluded because this will have a profound effect on treatment.

Hoarseness or alterations in voice have different causes depending on the age and social habits of the patient. A hoarse infant or child is more likely to have a congenital laryngeal abnormality, vocal nodules or laryngitis. An adolescent or young adult is more likely to have vocal nodules, laryngitis or benign tumours or polyps. Older adults who have a history of cigarette smoking and/or heavy alcohol intake are at risk from malignancy.

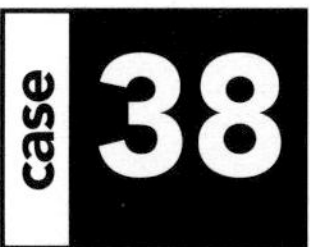

DIFFERENTIAL DIAGNOSIS

1. Angina
2. Anaemia
3. Coronary stenosis from thrombus formation

DISCUSSION

The patient seems to be describing classical symptoms of angina, namely characteristic chest pain precipitated by exertion. Angina is often worse after food because blood is diverted to the gut and on taking exercise in the cold because this causes skin vasoconstriction. A sudden worsening of angina symptoms may be the result of extra cardiac causes such as anaemia; more commonly it is caused by a sudden worsening of a coronary stenosis because of a thrombus developing on a cracked atheromatous plaque. This 'unstable' angina is more likely to lead to myocardial infarction.

There are no characteristic physical signs of angina caused by coronary artery disease, although a high blood pressure and signs of high plasma cholesterol should be sought.

The most characteristic feature of acute myocardial infarction, apart from severe and sustained chest pain, is massive reflex activation of the autonomic nervous system causing pallor, sweating and nausea. Ectopic beats under these conditions indicate increased myocardium irritability and may be a forerunner of ventricular fibrillation. Vasoconstriction tends to preserve the mean blood pressure but there is usually a narrow pulse pressure.

It is likely that the patient, who initially presented with unstable angina, is now in the process of have a myocardial infarct. The priorities are to give adequate analgesia, to transfer him somewhere where the cardiac rhythm can be monitored and ventricular fibrillation treated, and to arrange for treatment to restore patency to the blocked coronary artery.

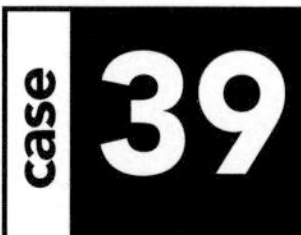

DIFFERENTIAL DIAGNOSIS

1. Left hemisphere ischaemic event
2. Left hemisphere haemorrhagic event

DISCUSSION

The episode 2 months previously appears to have been a transient ischaemic attack in the same arterial territory. Patients with a history of such events have a subsequent significant risk for further events or completed stroke in the same arterial territory.

The patient was right handed and dysphasic. The lesion was in the dominant (left) hemisphere in the middle cerebral (internal carotid) territory and was more likely to be ischaemic than haemorrhagic.

The patient had a nonfluent dysphasia with an impairment of grammar to the point where speech was often restricted to single words. Her comprehension was normal. The possibilities are either a Broca aphasia or a transcortical motor aphasia. The associated hemiparesis affecting both the arm and leg favours a Broca aphasia.

Ischaemic events in the carotid territory may be caused by small vessel occlusions associated with in-situ arterial degenerative disease (lacunes) or macroinfarcts which are almost always embolic in origin. If a cholesterol embolus was identified in this patient's left fundus, that would point to the likely mechanism of her stroke.

The most appropriate noninvasive procedure for assessment of the carotid bifurcation is duplex scanning. An alternative, noninvasive procedure, is magnetic resonance angiography. Only under certain circumstances would invasive angiography then be necessary.

If a stenosis exceeding 70% is found in the left carotid artery, the patient will be offered carotid endarterectomy. If there is a contralateral stenosis in the asymptomatic right carotid artery, there is as yet insufficient evidence to advise surgery on that artery. If the left carotid stenosis is less than 70%, the patient should be given antiplatelet therapy.

case 40

DIFFERENTIAL DIAGNOSIS

1. Bleeding oesophageal varices suggested by signs of liver disease and the history of alcohol
2. Peptic ulceration (gastric and duodenal) suggested by the history of associated pain, smoking and alcohol ingestion
3. Gastritis or duodenitis suggested by the history of nonsteroidal anti-inflammatory drug ingestion
4. Oesophagitis
5. Upper gastrointestinal neoplasia

DISCUSSION

Melena is a sign of bleeding from the oesophagus, stomach or duodenum and is caused by the effect of gastric acid on haemoglobin. Colonic bleeding does not cause melena.

This patient is hypovolaemic (tachycardic and hypotensive) and before the diagnosis can be elucidated he will require resuscitation.

There are three potential causes of upper gastrointestinal haemorrhage in this patient.

Firstly, the safe level of alcohol ingestion is approximately 28 units a week and patients often underestimate their alcohol consumption. There is a history of alcohol ingestion with evidence of liver cell damage from the jaundice, spider naevi and hepatomegaly. This suggests cirrhosis of the liver with portal hypertension, splenomegaly, ascites and formation of oesophageal varices. Variceal bleeding is usually brisk and may be catastrophic. Although melena may be a presenting feature, variceal haemorrhage is usually associated with both haematemesis and melena.

Secondly, the intermittent use of nonsteroidal anti-inflammatory drugs for analgesia puts the patient at risk of developing gastric and duodenal erosions and gastritis or duodenitis with upper gastrointestinal bleeding.

The third, and most likely, explanation of bleeding in this patient is a peptic ulcer. This is suggested by the concurrent upper abdominal discomfort. In patients with portal hypertension with oesophageal varices there is a high incidence of bleeding from concurrent duodenal ulceration. Duodenal ulcer symptoms are often relieved by drinking milk or simple antacids, however, in gastric ulceration, eating may aggravate symptoms.

Melena may also be the result of other causes from the oesophagus, stomach or duodenum. It may arise case 40

from oesophagitis (usually associated with heartburn and odynophagia), a benign or malignant neoplasm (usually associated with weight loss or vomiting) and a Mallory–Weiss tear (usually associated with retching that precedes a haematemesis).

The diagnosis may be confirmed, after the patient's resuscitation with appropriate fluids, by an upper gastrointestinal endoscopy.

case 41

DIFFERENTIAL DIAGNOSIS

1. Wernicke's encephalopathy

DISCUSSION

Your working diagnosis is Wernicke's encephalopathy. It is clear that the patient has drunk regularly in the past and probably more than he admitted to at the time of his medical a year before. His work pattern has deteriorated and he has begun to vomit. His gait has altered and he has had symptoms suggestive of a peripheral neuropathy. When giving the history, his short-term memory was defective, although at times spurious and apparently fictitious material was introduced.

His physical signs include hepatomegaly, bilateral cerebellar signs, bilateral sixth nerve palsies and changes in the lower limbs indicating a peripheral neuropathy. Wernicke's encephalopathy usually occurs in alcoholics, although it can be triggered by intractable vomiting. Often, patients have a combination of Wernicke's encephalopathy and Korsakov's psychosis, the latter suggested by the memory defect associated with confabulation. Many patients with Wernicke's encephalopathy have an associated peripheral neuropathy.

A blood film would more than likely to reveal evidence of a macrocytosis, whereas liver function tests would show abnormal enzyme levels, particularly gamma glutamyl transferase.

In some patients with Wernicke's encephalopathy, the brainstem or thalamic haemorrhages are sufficiently large to be detected by scanning. The scan may also reveal dilated cortical sulci but, with this length of history, is unlikely to show cerebellar atrophy.

Intravenous thiamine (vitamin B_1) should be started immediately. The patient would need life-long thiamine supplements. He has probably been drinking very heavily for 3 weeks and is likely to experience alcohol withdrawal effects. He would need intravenous heminevrin.

His memory may not recover. His nystagmus would resolve but not necessarily the sixth nerve palsies. He may well be left with residual cerebellar and neuropathic signs, even if he abstains from alcohol.

case 42

DIFFERENTIAL DIAGNOSIS

1. Ectopic beats
2. Coronary heart disease

DISCUSSION

The description in the history is very characteristic of ectopic beats. It is usually not possible clinically to distinguish between atrial and ventricular ectopics. The ectopic beat is not usually felt; it resets the cardiac cycle and causes a pause; the abnormally powerful next beat is what is felt by the patient. Ectopics tend to be more frequent and more readily noticed when the underlying heart rate is slow. This is why ectopics are often particularly troublesome when resting after effort, or at night, and why ß-blockers are often ineffective. Ectopic beats that are precipitated or made worse during exercise may be a feature of coronary heart disease but that is not the case here. Anxiety in itself will not precipitate ectopic beats but in someone who has ectopic beats the rise in adrenaline induced by anxiety can make them more frequent. The prevalence of ectopic beats rises progressively with age. In the absence of heart failure, valve disease or coronary disease, ectopic beats have a very benign prognosis. Drugs can induce ectopic beats either directly (e.g. digoxin, aminophylline) or by altering electrolyte balance. In this case the patient was found to have a low plasma potassium concentration which may have been caused by the bendrofluazide. Her electrocardiogram confirmed ventricular ectopics; an ambulatory electrocardiogram showed no other arrhythmia and echocardiography was normal.

case 43

DIFFERENTIAL DIAGNOSIS

1. Cerebellar stroke
   — infarct
   — haematoma

DISCUSSION

The patient has left-sided cerebellar signs with virtually no other abnormalities on examination at the time of admission. He has had a left cerebellar stroke that is clearly not haemorrhagic. A computerised tomography scan is almost always normal in the first few hours after a cerebral hemisphere or cerebellar hemisphere infarct. In the light of the patient's deterioration, he should be re-scanned. Probably either computerised tomography or magnetic resonance imaging scanning would be satisfactory because it is 4 days since the onset of his illness.

With the decline of the patient's conscious level he has developed additional physical signs. He appears to have a left sixth and seventh nerve palsy and the impairment of palatal elevation suggests there may well be bilateral tenth nerve palsies. In addition, he has developed bilateral extensor plantars. Cerebellar infarction, like cerebral infarction, is liable to be complicated by the development of oedema which appears within 2–3 days of onset. Swelling of the cerebellum can be accommodated by either downward or upward shift. Downward shift results in engagement of the cerebellar tonsils in the foramen magnum, upward shift results in compression of the brainstem and upward herniation through the tentorial notch. Probably both processes have occurred here.

Corticosteroids and osmotic diuretics will not exert any useful benefit. Ventriculo-atrial shunting will relieve any hydrocephalus secondary to fourth ventricular compression but will not deal with the primary pathology. It is preferable to perform decompression of the posterior fossa by excising the necrotic cerebellar tissue. The outcome is usually remarkably good.

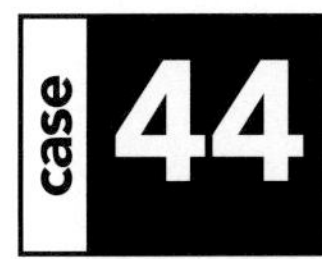

DIFFERENTIAL DIAGNOSIS

1. Left parietal skull fracture
2. Probable accidental injury

DISCUSSION

Any fracture in any child must trigger the following questions:

- How did this injury occur?
- Do the examination findings fit with the history supplied?
- Are there child protection issues that need to be shared with other agencies?

It is necessary to consider these issues even if they are at first less relevant than the immediate medical and surgical management. Many accidents are simply 'waiting to happen' and all healthcare professionals can become reluctant to consider a nonaccidental cause for a child's injuries.

If there are any doubts about these questions then the appropriate senior staff need to be involved as early as possible. It is essential to deal with issues logically and promptly, preferably following a local departmental protocol. Delays and inappropriate handling by less experienced staff can cause upset among the families concerned.

In the case of this baby, a thorough assessment of the history and an examination do not reveal any further factors to cause more concern about a nonaccidental injury. However, a senior colleague suggests admission, a cranial computerised tomography scan, ophthalmological assessment and liaison with the family's general practitioner and health visitor. The hospital social worker is informed of the admission.

Fundoscopy fails to demonstrate any evidence of retinal haemorrhages and the scan shows the fracture to be undisplaced without evidence of intracerebral haemorrhage or dural effusions.

The enquiries with health visitor and general practitioner do not reveal any concerns. The social worker says that the family are not known to local social services.

The senior paediatrician helps to give the results of the investigations to the family. He tells the family that this a fairly typical presentation of a parietal fracture. The injury is often over looked by the carers as the infant recovers quickly. There can be a delay of 24–48 h before the parietal swelling (a true cephalohaematoma) appears and presentation to a doctor occurs.

The paediatrician stresses the likelihood of an excellent outcome without long-term sequelae. A few minutes are spent addressing the guilty feelings that are inevitable when a momentary lapse in parenting can result in such a scenario. The father admits to feeling terrible since the fracture was diagnosed and both parents recognised that they had left her unattended on the bed for various lengths of time.

The baby is discharged home with follow-up arranged with the senior paediatrician.

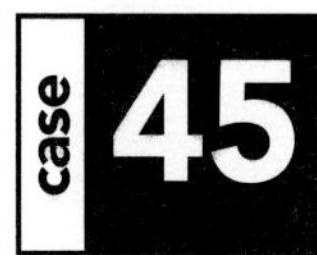

DIFFERENTIAL DIAGNOSIS

1. Asthma
2. Hyperventilation
3. Pulmonary embolism

DISCUSSION

The most likely diagnosis is asthma but there are a number of aspects of the history that need to be clarified. The history of intermittent wheezy breathlessness is virtually diagnostic of asthma and the question is whether this is still the diagnosis or whether something else has developed.

Features that suggest something new are the change in severity of the disease and the failure to control it as well as previously. In addition, there are two new symptoms, chest pain and light-headedness, neither of which are primary features of asthma.

On the other hand, the nocturnal wheeze and breathlessness is a very powerful pointer to asthma. It is common for asthmatics to complain bitterly about their sleep disturbance but appear normal by the next morning. The asthma may be out of control because the patient may be using the inhalers inadequately to provide maximum benefit.

Hyperventilation is suggested by the light-headedness. Patients may, in addition, have palpitations, tingling in the fingers or weakness in the legs. Breathlessness is usually at rest rather than on exertion and waking at night is unusual. Chest pain is often associated and is caused by the additional strain on the ribs and musculature. It can sometimes occur in patients with asthma and, when it does, the hyperventilation can make the asthma worse and the concomitant anxiety then makes the hyperventilation worse. The failure to reproduce the symptoms by a period of hyperventilation in the clinic is however a strong pointer against the diagnosis.

Pulmonary embolism is unlikely but should be considered because of its importance. Recurrent pleuritic pain and shortness of breath are the main features of recurrent small- or medium-sized emboli. Some episodes of haemoptysis are likely. In this patient there are no risk factors and the pain seems explicable by local chest wall tenderness.

Chronic obstructive lung disease is unlikely because the patient is too young, does not smoke and there is no sputum production.

The next stage is to ask the patient to do regular readings of peak flow and record the results. This should include any night-time episodes and the readings should be taken before having any bronchodilator treatment. It would be expected that this record would show recurrent 'dips' in the readings at night with partial recovery during the day. This would then confirm a diagnosis of asthma.

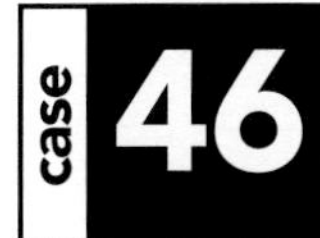

DIFFERENTIAL DIAGNOSIS

1. Gastric or duodenal ulcer suggested by site of pain, association with meals and relief with antacids
2. Gallstones suggested by right-sided abdominal pain, associated with meals in a well-nourished person
3. Pancreatitis suggested by epigastric pain related to meals in a heavy drinker
4. Nonulcerative dyspepsia suggested by the absence of any sinister features
5. Gastritis suggested by epigastric pain in a drinker or patient on nonsteroidal anti-inflammatory drugs

DISCUSSION

The recent onset of symptoms in this patient suggests an organic pathology.

The radiation of the pain to the right side of the abdomen in a plump person makes gallstone disease a possibility as does the exacerbation of the pain with meals. However, gallstones are more frequent in women and the discomfort is not usually relieved by antacids. Abdominal examination may reveal a positive Murphy's sign. An ultrasound examination of the biliary tree would reveal an acoustic shadow from the gallbladder confirming a gallstone.

The pain of pancreatitis usually radiates around the abdomen to the back and is exacerbated by lying flat and relieved by sitting forward. Pancreatitis may also associated with steatorrhoea. The two most common causes of pancreatitis are gallstones and alcohol ingestion. A plain abdominal radiograph or a computerised tomography scan of the abdomen would reveal calcification of the pancreas in chronic pancreatitis.

Gastritis and peptic ulcer pains are meal-related, may radiate to the right side of the abdomen and may be relieved with antacids. Duodenal ulcer pain occurs before meals and at night as opposed to gastric ulcer pain which is made worse by ingestion. The pain from a duodenal ulcer may radiate through to the back. An upper gastrointestinal endoscopy would be required to confirm the presence of a peptic ulcer or gastritis.

The pain from nonulcerative dyspepsia mimics the pain of a peptic ulcer, however, it is usually associated with bloating, nausea and early satiety and does not disturb the patient from his or her sleep. The endoscopy is normal in nonulcerative dyspepsia.

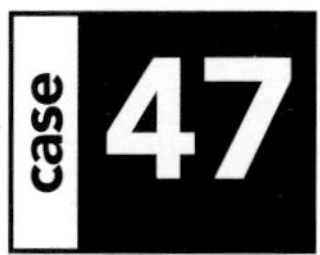

DIFFERENTIAL DIAGNOSIS

1. Central disc prolapse in the lumbosacral spine

DISCUSSION

The history is strongly suggestive of an acute disc prolapse. The bilateral distribution of the symptoms and signs and the evidence of sphincter disturbance suggests that this is a central rather than posterolateral prolapse. Plantar flexion (gastrocnemius and soleus) is supplied by L5 and S1 (mainly S1), knee flexion (hamstrings) by S1 and hip extension (gluteus maximus and medius) by S1. The posterior aspect of the thigh is supplied by S2 as is the inferior border of the buttock. The perianal area is supplied by sacral segments 3–5. The sensory deficit suggests, therefore, involvement of the sacral dermatomes from S2–S5.

This problem should be investigated as an emergency. Plain radiographs of the spine will not provide any useful data. The main alternatives are computerised tomography myelography or magnetic resonance imaging. The former is invasive but is generally more rapidly and widely available. The latter is the investigation of choice. It will allow assessment of all the lumbar spine rather than just the affected segment. A potential disadvantage occurs with computerised tomography myelography if the central disc prolapse (probably at L5/S1) is complete. Insufficient contrast may go past the obstruction to show the higher lumbar levels.

The only appropriate treatment here is surgical. The patient should be catheterised and taken to theatre immediately. Providing a satisfactory decompression of the cauda equina is achieved, the outlook should be good but further delay may well jeopardise this patient's recovery, particularly with regard to bladder function.

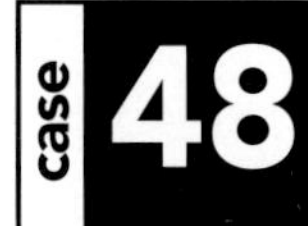

DIFFERENTIAL DIAGNOSIS

1. Pyloric obstruction suggested by absence of bile
2. Raised intracranial pressure suggested by occasional headache and morning vomiting
3. Drug therapy as digoxin toxicity can give rise to vomiting
4. Labyrinthitis which can give rise to vomiting

DISCUSSION

A history of recurrent upper abdominal pain that is worse during hunger and radiates through the back, suggests duodenal ulceration. Recurrent untreated duodenal ulceration may be complicated by pyloric stenosis. The pyloric stenosis, causes gastric outlet obstruction with distension of the stomach with gas and fluid giving rise to the 'succusion splash', has resulted in vomiting which has caused an aspiration pneumonia with right-sided chest signs in this patient. A malignant gastric neoplasm causing pyloric obstruction should also be considered despite a history of classical duodenal ulceration.

Large bowel obstruction usually gives rise to faeculent vomiting, absolute constipation, colicky abdominal pain and abdominal distension. Large bowel obstruction can therefore be excluded from the differential diagnosis.

The vomiting with raised intracranial pressure is worse in the morning; the headaches are also worse on awakening. However, there are no signs of raised intracranial pressure such as papilloedema, enlargement of the blind spot and loss of the peripheral visual fields.

Digoxin toxicity may occur, particularly with renal impairment and can give rise to vomiting but bile is usually not absent.

Other causes of vomiting such as biliary tract disorders, metabolic disorders and psychological disorders such as anorexia nervosa and bulimia are not likely in this case.

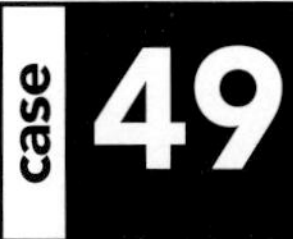

DIFFERENTIAL DIAGNOSIS

1. Lateral popliteal palsy
2. L4 radiculopathy

DISCUSSION

The motor impairment was in the distribution of the lateral popliteal nerve. Often, with such lesions, extensor hallucis longus is the most severely affected muscle and sensory changes tend to be inconspicuous. The ankle jerk would be normal in such cases. Although there was a long history of back pain, that pain had never had any radicular components and the motor findings detailed could not be explained by a single nerve root lesion. The patient was known to be anxious and perhaps slightly depressed but it was clear that his problem was organically determined.

The lateral popliteal nerve is particularly susceptible to trauma as it winds round the neck of the fibula. It is likely that that was where the lesion was situated. The nerve can be damaged by fractures, by prolonged pressure on the nerve because of immobility (e.g. in a postoperative patient) and also by prolonged kneeling, as here. The nerve can also be affected by any of the conditions capable of damaging the vasa nervorum, for example, diabetes or polyarteritis nodosa, but there was no evidence for such a problem here. You should look for a positive Tinel's sign at the neck of the fibula, where the nerve can be readily palpated. A positive sign would strongly support your assumption that that was the site of the lesion.

Electromyography and particularly nerve conduction studies should be most helpful. It was too early to detect denervation in the affected muscles but you would expect to demonstrate a depressed or absent lateral popliteal nerve action potential at the neck of the fibula and you should be looking to demonstrate a slowing of motor conduction across the presumed site of damage at that level.

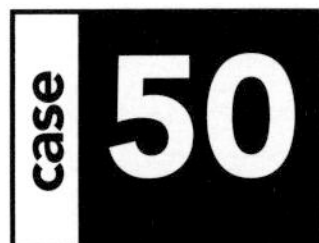

DIFFERENTIAL DIAGNOSIS

1. Heart block from Stokes–Adams attack
2. Ventricular tachycardia
3. Postural hypotension
4. Vertebrobasilar insufficiency

DISCUSSION

Blackouts in elderly people usually have a cardiac rather than a primary neurological cause. The differential diagnosis would include heart block (Stokes–Adams attack) a fast arrhythmia such as ventricular tachycardia, postural hypotension or vertebrobasilar insufficiency. The observation that the patient goes pale during an attack and turns pink on recovery strongly suggests a cardiac cause such as complete heart block. Important features to look out for on examination include the pulse rate and rhythm, the lying and standing blood pressure, the presence of heart murmurs and whether any bruits can be heard over the neck.

On examination the striking feature is the slow pulse rate. A slow pulse is uncommon at this age and nearly always means a problem with the cardiac conducting system and/or drug intoxication. Atenolol causes pulse slowing, it is also mainly excreted by the kidneys and often accumulates to toxic levels in elderly patients. The patient also has carotid sinus hypersensitivity which may be contributing to her symptoms. She does not have postural hypotension. There is a soft systolic murmur but nothing else to suggest aortic disease. At this age, calcium deposits in and around the aortic valve are common and may also interfere with conduction.

Her electrocardiogram showed complete heart block. After stopping the atenolol she felt better but a 24-h electrocardiogram cable still showed episodes of heart block and she was fitted with a pacemaker. Echocardiography showed calcification around the aortic valve.

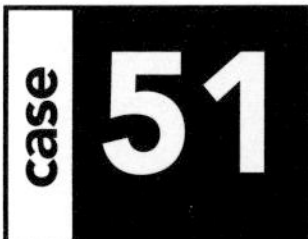

DIFFERENTIAL DIAGNOSIS:

1. Acute optic neuritis
2. Retinal detachment
3. Central serous retinopathy

DISCUSSION

This patient has had an attack of optic neuritis. Prodromal pain is very characteristic and is typically worsened by ocular movement. The visual impairment predominates centrally but varies in severity. An afferent pupillary defect is almost inevitable in this situation. Where the inflammatory process is close to the optic nerve head, disc swelling ensues and may be associated with peripapillary haemorrhages. The majority of patients recover from optic neuritis. There is nothing in the history to suggest a retinal disorder, for example, retinal detachment or central serous retinopathy. The symptoms a year previously suggest a cervical cord lesion at that time.

The abdominal responses should be present in a woman of this age group. Two to three beats of symmetrical ankle clonus is a normal finding.

The working diagnosis is multiple sclerosis. The history of transient sensory disturbance a year before is significant. Lhermitte's sign can occur in other conditions but, in a young person without a history of neck trauma, is strongly suggestive of multiple sclerosis. The relative paucity of neurological signs at this point does not refute the diagnosis.

Magnetic resonance imaging is the investigation of choice here. Almost all patients with multiple sclerosis will be expected to have areas of abnormal signal which typically tend to be periventricular. Lesions within the corpus callosum are particularly characteristic. If you decide to proceed to cerebrospinal fluid examination, your attention should focus on measuring the immunoglobulin G ratios and looking for oligoclonal bands. An abnormal immunoglobulin G index (comparing the immunoglobulin G/albumin ratio in cerebrospinal fluid to that in the serum) is abnormal in approximately 70% of multiple sclerosis patients. Oligoclonal bands that are not duplicated by comparable bands in the serum are found in approximately 90% of definite multiple sclerosis patients.

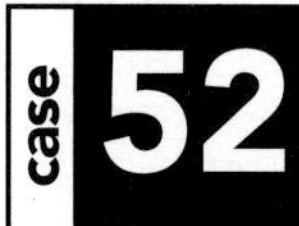

DIFFERENTIAL DIAGNOSIS

1. Cancer of large bowel suggested by *S bovis* endocarditis and hard liver
2. Polyp of large bowel
3. Infective diarrhoea due to travel abroad
4. Antibiotic-related diarrhoea due to a long course of antibiotics for septicaemia
5. Ulcerative colitis that presents with diarrhoea and rectal bleeding
6. Diverticulosis that can present with diarrhoea and brisk rectal bleeding

DISCUSSION

Blood in stools indicates that the disorder is caused by an organic pathology and excludes a functional cause for the symptoms.

S bovis septicaemia is associated with large bowel neoplasm, benign or malignant. In the presence of rectal bleeding and diarrhoea, bowel neoplasm must be the most likely cause of this patient's symptoms. In association with the hard, irregular liver, he probably has a colonic neoplasm with liver metastases. The causes of hard knobbly liver include malignancy, macronodular cirrhosis and polycystic liver disease. Some form of lower gastrointestinal imaging (colonoscopy or barium enema) is mandatory with his symptoms.

Clostridium difficile and some other infections, such as amoebiasis, salmonella, shigella and campylobacter, can present with bloody diarrhoea but *C difficile* is very unusual 9 months after the administration of antibiotics. Infective diarrhoea is a good second differential in view of the foreign travel history. A stool sample should be sent for microbiological analysis and should also be tested for *C difficile* toxin.

The presence of normal appearance on a rigid sigmoidoscopy would exclude ulcerative colitis which always affects the rectum and presents with bloody diarrhoea, tenesmus and crampy abdominal pain.

Proctoscopy, although normal here, should always be followed with an examination of the remaining large intestine even in the presence of haemorrhoids to exclude a neoplasm higher up in the colon.

Diverticulosis, usually presenting with left-sided abdominal pain and a change in bowel habit, is unlikely to give rise to hepatomegaly unless complicated by abscess formation. However, this is unlikely as the patient is not febrile. The bleeding from diverticulosis is usually very brisk and often results in urgent admission to hospital.

case 53

DIFFERENTIAL DIAGNOSIS

1. Cor pulmonale from chronic obstructive airways disease

DISCUSSION

Heart failure is not a diagnosis but a collation of symptoms and signs. In this patient, insufficient thought has been given to the nature and cause of the heart failure. The long history before presentation makes left ventricular failure less likely and this and the heavy smoking history, together with the productive cough, suggest that the breathlessness is on the basis of chronic airways obstruction. The failure of the breathlessness to respond to diuretics also suggests an alternative cause. Many patients with chronic airways obstruction are unable to breath lying flat.

The cardiovascular signs are all of right ventricular failure and indeed indicate the development of tricuspid regurgitation as a result. The failure to locate the apex beat suggests that the left ventricle is not involved or that hyperinflated lungs are interposed between the chest wall and heart. The respiratory signs are compatible with airways disease and a few coarse basal crackles should not be equated with the profuse fine late crackles of pulmonary oedema. The likely sequence of events is slow progression of fixed airways obstruction over a number of years with the development of hypoxia. This has led to pulmonary hypertension and right heart failure or cor pulmonale. She probably has carbon dioxide retention and the delivery of an efficient oxygen supply during the examination has led to the development of carbon dioxide narcosis. Further assessment should include a chest radiograph (which will show cardiomegaly but not pulmonary oedema), arterial blood gases and spirometry.

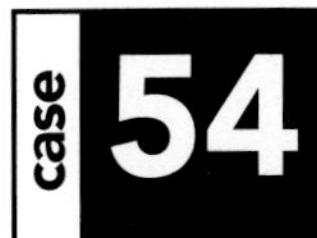

DIFFERENTIAL DIAGNOSIS

1. Sarcoidosis caused by fever in a young woman with symptoms and signs of pulmonary fibrosis
2. Drugs: penicillin or the oral contraceptive pill
3. Inflammatory bowel disease due to a family history of psoriasis (human lymphocyte antigen B27-related) and history of loose stools
4. Infections such as salmonella and campylobacter

DISCUSSION

The history of this patient's symptoms predates the administration of penicillin, therefore, although this drug could give rise to erythema nodosum, it is not likely to do so in this case.

The history of loose stools and erythema nodosum would fit with an inflammatory or infective bowel pathology, however, this cannot be associated with the pulmonary findings and is therefore unlikely.

Sarcoidosis can give rise to noncasaeting granulomatous involvement of the lungs and large intestine and results in fever as well as erythema nodosum and diarrhoea. The diagnosis is particularly likely in a young woman presenting with erythema nodosum and respiratory symptoms suggestive of pulmonary sarcoidosis.

Other causes of erythema nodosum such as tuberculosis, leprosy, deep fungal infection, pregnancy, Beçhet's disease are unlikely. Between 20 and 40% of cases of erythema nodosum remain idiopathic. The diagnosis of sacroidosis is made on history, examination, chest radiograph (shows enlarged hilar lymph nodes) and a positive Kveim test.

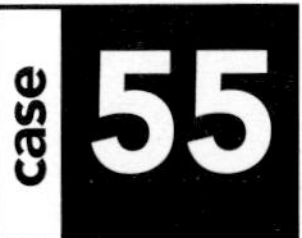

DIFFERENTIAL DIAGNOSIS

1. Ramsay Hunt syndrome
2. Bell's palsy
3. Other causes of a lower motor neuron facial weakness

DISCUSSION

This patient has a lower motor neuron facial paresis. He was aware of substantial weakness of orbicularis oculi (the eye is not closing adequately) as well as of the lower face (he is dribbling from the angle of his mouth). The global impairment of motor function on the left side was confirmed on physical examination. Branches of the facial nerve include the greater superficial petrosal nerve, the nerve to stapedius and the chorda tympani. Assessment of lachrymation in patients with facial palsy is difficult but the hyperacusis and the loss of taste indicate that the lesion in this case was proximal both to the exit of the nerve to stapedius and the exit of the chorda tympani.

The presence of a rash raises the possibility of herpetic infection. In the Ramsay Hunt syndrome, the lower motor neuron facial weakness results from herpetic infection of the geniculate ganglion. A vesicular rash may be detectable over part of the pinna, the palate or the tonsillar region. Scab formation ensues. Many patients with the Ramsay Hunt syndrome will have a lymphocytic pleocytosis in the cerebrospinal fluid despite the lack of any evidence of a more diffuse meningoencephalitic picture.

There is clearly impairment of eye closure and the presence of scleral infection indicates that the cornea is at risk from damage. The patient should be instructed not to touch the eye and should wear a soft eye pad at night. The eye should be kept lubricated with artificial tears. If signs of corneal damage emerge, the eye will need protection by a lateral tarsorrhaphy. The outcome of the Ramsay Hunt syndrome is probably no different from the outcome of Bell's palsy. Some 80% of patients will make a full recovery. Incomplete recovery in the remainder may be accompanied by signs of aberrant reinnervation.

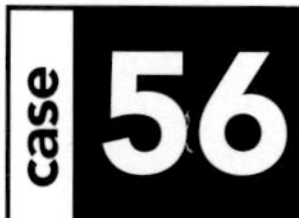

DIFFERENTIAL DIAGNOSIS

1. Hypothyroidism suggested by tiredness and slow relaxing reflexes
2. Hyperprolactinaemia suggested by increased breast secretions
3. Adrenocorticotrophic hormone deficiency suggested by pallor, weakness and postural hypotension
4. Diabetes suggested by increased micturition

DISCUSSION

She has multiple deficiencies of the endocrine glands. There is suppression of the thyroid axis with tiredness, lethargy, constipation and slow relaxing reflexes. There is suppression of the adrenal axis with weakness, pallor and postural hypotension. There is a deficiency in gonadotrophins with amenorrhoea and loss of axillary and pubic hair. There is a reduction in antidiuretic hormone production with polyuria. In addition, there is hyperprolactinaemia with galactorrhoea.

All these symptoms and signs point to hypopituitarism. Whereas in primary adrenal failure (Addison's disease) the skin becomes pigmented, in hypopituitarism there is loss of melanin from the skin, resulting in pallor. In postpartum hypopituitarism, lactation fails to establish because of the failure to release prolactin. The most likely cause in this lady is hypotension occurring during labour that would have caused pituitary infarction (Sheehan's syndrome).

Other causes of hypopituitarism such as pituitary tumours, both primary and secondary, are not likely as they usually present with raised intracranial pressure or compression of the optic chaism. There are no symptoms or signs to suggest raised intracranial pressure such as early morning headache, vomiting, papilloedema, enlargement of the blind spot or loss of the peripheral visual fields. Compression of the optic chiasm would result in bitemporal hemianopia.

Hypopituitarism may also result from infectious disease such as tuberculosis and sarcoidosis and iatrogenic disorders such as previous surgery or radiotherapy but that is not likely in this woman.

case 57

DIFFERENTIAL DIAGNOSIS

1. Rheumatoid arthritis
2. Systemic lupus erythematosus (SLE)
3. Psoriatic arthropathy

DISCUSSION

The history strongly supports the diagnosis of organic disease. Although the patient had been stressed and appeared anxious during the examination, the symptoms point to an arthropathy of some sort. The concept of repetitive strain injury is a nebulous one and is hardly likely to explain such a symmetrical picture. Furthermore, although her symptoms had improved after leaving work (coinciding with her pregnancy) they had become considerably worse after the delivery of her child. The pattern of involvement, based on the history and the early morning stiffness, is suggestive of rheumatoid arthritis; the diagnosis is supported by the results of the examination. The changes in mobility of the right elbow and left wrist are characteristic, as are the findings in the finger joints. There are no systemic features to suggest SLE and the distribution of the joint changes is not that of psoriatic arthropathy.

Both the C-reactive protein and the erythrocyte sedimentation rate should be measured. Both, particularly the latter, may be normal at this stage of the disease. An elevated titre of rheumatoid factor, however, would strongly support the diagnosis of rheumatoid arthritis. Radiographs should be taken, although it must be appreciated that it takes about 6 months before rheumatoid synovitis results in radiographically visible erosions.

Important issues in management include patient education, a programme of regular exercises and drug control of symptoms and inflammation. Nonsteroidal anti-inflammatory drugs are the cornerstone of initial treatment.

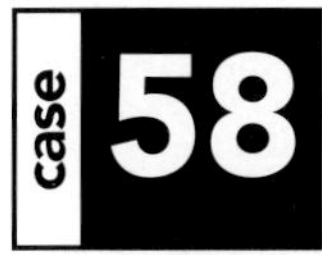

DIFFERENTIAL DIAGNOSIS

1. Heart failure
2. Chronic lung disease
3. Anaemia due to aspirin

DISCUSSION

There are four possible causes of breathlessness that should be considered as a result of the patient's history. (It is possible to grade shortness of breath according to activity precipitating the symptoms.)

The patient has ischaemic heart disease that might, in itself, cause breathlessness or be associated with left-sided heart failure. A history of angina orthopnoea and paroxysmal nocturnal dyspnoea would usually be present in cardiac breathlessness.

The patient had smoked for 30 years and a history of wheezing, coughing and productive sputum would often accompany a pulmonary cause of breathlessness.

Recurrent pulmonary embolism may cause shortness of breath and may occur in the absence of coughing up blood. The patient usually presents acutely and may be associated with symptoms of right heart failure or show electrocardiographic evidence of right heart strain. There may also be an obvious predisposing factor usually related to a period of abnormal immobilisation.

The introduction of aspirin 6 months previously raises a possibility of anaemia and a story of indigestion or black stools would address this possibility. The likely diagnosis is clarified by the examination in which the striking physical sign was conjunctival pallor. There was no evidence of significant heart or lung disease. The brachycardia was associated with the ß-blocker and the soft murmur was not associated with left ventricular hypertrophy (hyperdynamic or displaced apex beat) or radiation of the murmur to the carotids. The most likely diagnosis is breathlessness caused by progressive anaemia which in turn was caused by chronic aspirin ingestion. This usually presents as an iron deficiency anaemia and is normally associated with occult bleeding. Low-dose aspirin causes gastrointestinal blood loss or, by virtue of its antiplatelet effect, might stimulate blood loss from an alimentary tract disorder such as a silent peptic ulcer, colonic polyps or cancer and vascular abnormalities such as angiodysplasia.